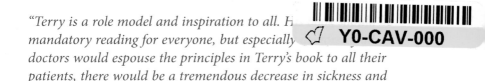

"Terry is a role model and inspiration to all. H... mandatory reading for everyone, but especially ... doctors would espouse the principles in Terry's book to all their patients, there would be a tremendous decrease in sickness and disease and a huge increase in the quality of everyone's life."

Jan McBarron, M.D.

"Terry is a true pioneer and thought leader on the cutting edge of natural research. Want to know what natural treatments will be wildly popular in 10-20 years? Simply see what Terry is using NOW!"

Jacob Teitelbaum MD, author of Real Cause, Real Cure, From Fatigued to Fantastic! and the popular Cures A-Z iPhone/Droid app

"Terry Lemerond is one of the most knowledgeable people I've ever had the pleasure of working with. His passion for health and vitality is exceeded only by his knowledge, wisdom and compassion. A true original!"

Jonny Bowden, PhD, CNS aka "The Rogue Nutritionist", author of The 150 Healthiest Foods on Earth and The Great Cholesterol Myth

"Terry Lemerond has written a book which belongs in the hands of every person who wants to know how to enjoy life to the fullest."

Robert C. Martin, D.C., Clinical Nutritionist, National Syndicated Host of Health Talk

"Terry is my mentor and my idol. He is one of the most passionate, knowledgeable figures in the natural health arena. He not only writes, talks about and loves vibrant health...he LIVES it!"

Holly Lucille, ND, expert, author, and host of Myth Defyers with Dr. Holly on Veria cable network

"Terry Lemerond is one of the greats in the natural health scene for all the right reasons. He combines seemingly boundless passion with dedication, a lot of valuable knowledge, and the consistency that comes from walking his talk. Terry is an inspiration. When it comes to vibrant health, he knows exactly what he's talking about. Read and learn."

Chris Kilham, Medicine Hunter

"Terry Lemerond is the most healthy, energetic, positive and spiritually sound person I know. Read this book and learn how he does it."

Siri Khalsa, Editor of Nutrition News

"As you go through life, many decisions you make will affect your health. In Seven Keys to Vibrant Health, *Terry Lemerond teaches you how to live your life in a manner that will maximize your potential for wellness. This is a book that can change your life for the better—not only by keeping you healthy, but also by showing you how you can live a life of personal fulfillment."*

Melvyn R. Werbach, M.D.

"Terry is that rarest of individuals—his expertise in natural medicine is matched only by his extraordinary compassion and generosity. His work in health and wellness has improved the lives of millions of people, and Seven Keys to Vibrant Health *has captured his philosophy in a comprehensive "owner's manual" for the human body!"*

Cheryl Myers, R.N., B.A., Author and Integrative Health Nurse

*"*Seven Keys to Vibrant Health *is a landmark, a guidepost! It provides the reader with a simple method to live a healthier, happier, longer, more pain-free life. Each chapter is a jewel. I found myself going back to the book, over and over again."*

Anthony J. Cichoke, M.A., D.C., D.A.C.B.N.

"…must-read for every household…"

Earl Mindell, Ph.D., *author of* The Vitamin Bible

"Terry Lemerond is a gentleman, a scholar, and an altruist. His book is an invaluable collection of scientifically proven tips on extending the quality and quantity of life while preventing and even reversing disease. America would spring into a new era of wellness and prosperity if these principles were adopted."

Patrick Quillin, Ph.D., R.D., CNS, *author of 8 books and Vice President of Nutrition for Cancer Treatment Centers of America*

Seven Keys to Vibrant Health

by

Terry Lemerond

www.TerryTalksNutrition.com

Disease is Nature Out of Balance

Cover design by: *Jill Baker*
Photography by: *Steve Eliasen*
Copyediting by: *Jennifer Hansgate*
Production by: *Jill Baker*

Library of Congress Catalog Card Number: 99-71238
ISBN 978-1-62620-167-5

PRINTED IN THE UNITED STATES OF AMERICA

Dedication

This book is dedicated to my loving family:
Brad, Stephanie, Roman and Angelique Lemerond;
Teppie, Matt, Anna and Clare Schueller;
and especially my wife, Debra.

Through Jesus Christ and His Divine Mercy, I know all things are possible.

TABLE OF CONTENTS

Acknowledgments

I would like to express my love and gratitude to the many people who offered their guidance, encouragement, valuable support, and friendship over the years that I developed and refined my personal health beliefs.

My thanks go to you, the reader, for opening this book to learn more about natural health. I hope your journey is enlightening and that you will share the message of healthy living with those around you. I could ask for no greater reward.

But most important of all, I thank God for His guidance and blessings, for He has always been the center of my life, both personally and in business. This book and my journey could not have been possible without the love and care I feel from God. I cannot claim to have the skills or the talents to take credit for the success that has blessed my life. Truly, God has touched me in a way that I can only praise and thank Him for every day of my life.

PREFACE TO THE REVISED EDITION

In the time since *Seven Keys to Vibrant Health* was first published, my thinking on diet and exercise has undergone changes. I am an avid reader and student of health-related research, and I continually adjust my life plan as I learn about new techniques and ideas for optimal health. I realized it was time that this book was updated to include the changes I have made in my own diet, exercise and supplement routines. However, the original inspiration for this book remains the same—to bring to you, the reader, the knowledge that you can make lasting changes for better health in your own life, as I have in mine.

PREFACE

Dear Reader:

The reason I decided to write this book is to share an insight that took me *years* to discover for myself: We can choose the kind of lives we want to live. When we start making conscious choices about our spirituality, attitude, relationships, lifestyle habits, exercise, diet, and supplementation— we come closer to achieving vibrant health and enduring happiness.

Why should you listen to me? After all, I'm not a doctor or a psychologist or even a professional writer. I was not born into wealth or privilege; I was not blessed with extraordinary genius. What I do have is a lifelong passion for natural health and self-empowerment. I don't believe our health and our lives are determined for us—I believe we make choices that determine what they will be.

It isn't easy. Change means giving up familiar ways of thinking and eating and interacting with others. And you've got a lot to lose: a negative attitude, loneliness, hopelessness, bad habits, fatigue, and poor health. Of course, if you feel you'd be better off without these things, then maybe you're ready for change. I can promise you that once you make these changes, you'll never look back.

Your human body is not just flesh and bones. It responds to your thoughts, your environment, your food choices, your spirit, your emotions. We are in a constant, complex, dynamic relationship with the world. When you work on each important area of your life, you'll find they work together to create a greater whole. For example, when you exercise, you improve your mood, which fosters a more positive attitude. When you develop meaningful relationships, you are more motivated to take care of your body through a healthful diet. They are all interrelated; and as one area unfolds, it touches and enriches every other area of your life.

My company has enjoyed great success with nutritional and botanical supplements and natural medicines. But I didn't get into this business because I was interested in making money. I chose natural health because it is my passion and I want people like you to enjoy extraordinary health, and perhaps more importantly, I want you to realize you can do it for yourself.

By opening this book, you have just taken an important step. May God bless you with health, prosperity, and success.

Terry

Terry Lemerond

INTRODUCTION

Seven Keys to Vibrant Health provides a blueprint for health that I have seen work miracles in my life and the lives of others. I did not "discover" these keys; people who are truly healthy simply possess these traits. My belief is that if you or I can also possess these keys, we too, can achieve optimal health and a better life.

Your life will improve if you follow the guidelines described in this book. No matter where you are in life—old or young, rich or poor, no matter what your personal history or education level—you can always get better from the moment you decide to improve. Making the decision to get better is the number one step to a life filled with more health, happiness, passion, and joy.

As is the case in achieving anything we desire, we first have to decide what it is that we truly want. Do you really want to have better health? How would you feel if you possessed vibrant, radiant health and energy? Once we really become focused on what it is we want, the next steps involve unlocking the keys to achieve our goal.

The farmer can decide to plant the seed, but before he plants, he must have some tools. He has to cultivate the land, he has to till and fertilize the soil. He must do many things to prepare the earth before he plants the seed.

Planting an idea or goal in a human being is a similar process. We can't just plant the seed. We must use the right tools to cultivate it, to nurture the seed so it will grow. Those tools come in the form of patience, faith, and tenacity; of perseverance when we fear the seed won't germinate. The farmer, when he plants the seed, doesn't sit and fret and worry that the seed isn't going to come up. He knows from past experience that, without some unforeseen natural catastrophe, a properly nurtured seed will germinate.

I've learned over the years that the same scenario applies to the human experience. The seed of a goal or dream will germinate, but we need to have the faith, the patience, the tenacity, and the perseverance to believe it will grow and just work in good faith.

So many times, I have seen people give up on their goals or dreams, especially regarding health, before they have really given them a chance. They lose faith. I like to tell people the story of the bamboo tree because it is such a beautiful example of the power of diligence.

A village received a seed of the bamboo tree as a gift from a neighboring village. They were told to plant it, water it, and care for it, so it would grow to a great size and provide shade from the hot sun for the village.

The villagers planted the seed and cared for it for one full year, but nothing happened. Many of the villagers wanted to give up. "Why should we work so hard to care for this seed when it is obvious that it is dead and will never grow?" one of them asked the chief of the village. The chief, a man of great faith, trusted the seed would eventually grow to a great bamboo tree. He was able to paint the picture in the minds of all the villagers of how magnificent it would be when the bamboo tree reached maturity. Because of the power of his faith and vision, the villagers continued to work hard, despite the fact that nothing happened for over four years. Finally, during the fifth year, a sprout started to come through the soil. A miracle was proclaimed when, just 90 days after the first sprout, the chief's vision—a ninety-foot bamboo tree—became a reality.

Why did it take five years before any evidence appeared that the seed had germinated? While nothing was apparent above the ground, under the ground a very extensive root system was developing to provide the kind of support that would allow the bamboo shoots to grow at an amazing rate— a foot a day. In order to support such incredible growth, the seed, in all its wisdom, was growing downward, rather than upward to form the huge foundation of root systems necessary to reach for the sun.

To achieve good health, you too, must develop a strong foundation. This takes time. Many people with whom I have come into contact believe that, after abusing themselves for 20-30 years, they can simply take a bottle of vitamins for a month, put together some sort of health or nutritional program, go on a weight-loss program, or exercise for a couple of weeks, and reverse all the years of abuse. When they don't see an obvious improvement after a month or so, they become discouraged and quit. What they don't realize is that they're building a strong foundation. If they persevere, once they reach a certain point, it's just like the bamboo tree: growth is exponential.

The human body is constantly regenerating. Because the cells in our bodies are continually changing, we can create a whole new self over time. For example, every three to four days, we gain a whole new lining in the gastrointestinal tract as new cells are formed to replace damaged old cells. In just thirty days, we renew our entire skin, and every six weeks, we make an entirely new liver. We live within the most amazing piece of machinery. (I don't like the word machinery, but use it for lack of a better word.) We can be very abusive to our bodies, yet they are very forgiving. If you give your body enough time, you can actually recreate your entire system.

So often I see people start a new health or weight-loss program but then give up far too early. Don't give up. I have seen the *Seven Keys to Vibrant Health* work wonders in my own life. Follow these keys, and you will achieve a healthier life. Believe it, because it is true.

My Journey to a Vibrant, Healthy Life

When I was growing up, I was fortunate (or unfortunate) to have access to many things that weren't good for me. Junk food, candies, and soft drinks became the major staples of my diet. As a young man of 20, I weighed over 200 pounds. At a height of 5'6", I was nearly as wide around as I was tall. In addition to being fat, I also had very severe hypoglycemia which resulted in a lot of mental, emotional, and behavioral problems due to the severe mood swings caused by my erratically plummeting blood sugar levels.

Because of my unruly behavior and attitude, I was not a very well-liked person. I knew my life was in trouble, so I joined the Marine Corps. I wanted to see if they could "make a man out of me." Joining the Marine Corps definitely changed my life for the better. Perhaps the best thing that happened to me was meeting Captain Ed Vito, who helped me learn the value of good health and proper nutrition.

I met Captain Vito when I joined the weight-lifting team after boot camp. I had lost a lot of weight during boot camp—a side effect of twelve weeks of continuous calisthenics, obstacle courses, marching, and running. I was definitely in better shape, but didn't have good muscle tone, so I joined the weight-lifting team.

Captain Vito was knowledgeable not only about weight-lifting but also about nutrition. I was very fortunate to be taken under his wing and introduced to the tremendous value of proper nutrition. When he took me home on weekends, I saw the healthful diet he and his family ate. Their diet focused on fresh fruits and vegetables, whole grains, sprouts, and a lot of other foods I had never eaten before.

In 1959, Captain Vito also took me to a health food store for the very first time—a small store in Oceanside, California. At that time, health food stores were much smaller than they are today. There were few products on the shelves, but a lot more than I had ever seen.

With Captain Vito's introduction, I became completely fascinated with health. I noticed that as I became healthier, I became much happier. My mood swings disappeared, and I felt better about life than I ever had. As my muscle tone improved, I looked healthier than I ever had. When I returned to Green Bay in 1962 after my stint in the Marines, people didn't recognize the man I had become.

I was extremely excited about what healthy food, good nutrition, and vitamins could do. When I left, Green Bay had no health food stores, so I was delighted when I looked in the *Yellow Pages* to discover that a store called Bay Natural Foods had recently opened. Immediately, I went down and introduced myself to the owner, Claire Delsmann. A delightful lady who had never married, Claire built the store by treating her customers like family.

Eventually, the store grew until it became too much for Claire to handle alone. I found myself helping her out for free before I went to work and on weekends, because I loved the store and was so glad it was available in Green Bay. I was working nights at a machine shop but would drop by the store in the morning just to say hello. I worked for Claire for about seven years, part-time, for free. I ran the store for her when she was on vacation. When she took a day off, I'd come in at 9:00 a.m. and work until a couple of minutes to 3:00 p.m., then run across town to the machine shop.

Finally, in 1969, Claire just couldn't run the store anymore. She had to sell but wanted somebody who shared her philosophy and would continue to run it like an extended family. This store was Claire's "baby." She wanted to make sure it was loved and nurtured.

Claire knew how much I loved the store. I was there all the time. When you love someone, you want to be there, you want to touch them, you want to hold them, you want to know everything that you can about them. Strange as it may sound, this was the kind of love I had for Bay Natural Foods. So, I was there all the time. I would stop in before work, after work, in between, any time I had a chance, I would go to help Claire or to read.

Claire wanted someone with that kind of dedication to take over the store, but I didn't have the money, so selling to me just didn't make sense. Finally, she found a person who had the money and wanted to buy the store, but she wasn't comfortable selling to a stranger. So, on a Saturday afternoon in February 1969, the course of my life changed forever.

Claire usually closed the store at noon on Saturdays. On this particular Saturday, however, I was staying late to paint the walls and spruce the store up a bit. Claire began telling me her dreams and what she wanted to see happen to the store. When I replied, "That's great. I support you 100%. I want that to happen for you, and I hope it does," she said, "Well, it can, if someone buys the store that has the same philosophy I have." When I said, "I agree with you completely," she asked, "Terry, why don't you buy the store?"

I explained to Claire that although owning Bay Natural Foods would be a dream come true, I didn't have any money. I couldn't see how it would be possible on my machine shop wages. Claire's desire for me to buy the store was so great, she decided to help me. With Claire's help, as well as some help from my mother and the bank, I was able to raise enough cash to buy the store.

From 1969 to 1981, I worked in Bay Natural Foods, educating people about the value of good nutrition and proper nutritional supplementation. Through years of study and experience, I had learned that certain vitamins, minerals, herbs, and glandular concentrates would produce far better results when combined than when they were taken individually. Rather than sending people home with a dozen different bottles of supplements, I wanted to use formulas that *combined* the essential nutrients necessary to meet my clients' specific nutritional needs. I had a dream: a company that would develop and sell state-of-the-art nutritional and botanical products designed to support specific body functions. In 1981, I started a company called Enzymatic Therapy®.

Like the bamboo tree, this company shot to the heights after a proper germination. While there, I introduced some important firsts to the U.S. health food market, including the concept of botanical standardization, glucosamine sulfate, standardized *Ginkgo biloba*, saw palmetto extract, enteric coated peppermint oil and IP-6.

After almost 20 years of running this company, during which the formula line expanded dramatically, I decided it was time to move on to new things. I sold Enzymatic Therapy (which is still in business today under its new ownership). However, I could not walk away from the industry entirely, as I had too much passion for the people and products I was still encountering every day. I dedicated time to helping others improve their natural products, and to introducing important European researchers with interesting innovations to quality companies in the United States. I was something of a match-maker!

Although I enjoyed working with researchers around the world, I realized I was no longer perfectly aligned with my dream. I missed creating my own products; I missed having a direct connection to my dearest home: the health food retail industry. So a little over 5 years ago, I founded a new company, called EuroPharma®, and introduced the *Terry Naturally*® line of products, which includes the award winning natural pain reliever, Curamin®.

Like the bamboo tree, EuroPharma took time to establish its roots, but patience has paid off. As a result of a commitment to providing the absolute best products, EuroPharma has established itself as the leader in the industry. I am so proud of how much our company has grown and expanded. We are now available in all 50 states and several foreign countries, and our product line has grown to over 100 supplements and natural medicines.

The growth and success of EuroPharma is based on the company's adherence to the same keys which are detailed in this book.

I hope you enjoy *Seven Keys to Vibrant Health*. I pray that it will answer some of your questions about health and will help inspire you to lead a life filled with vibrant health and happiness.

Terry Lemerond
Terry Talks Nutrition

CHAPTER ONE

KEY #1—SPIRITUALITY

STEP 1
Realize the power of prayer

STEP 2
Make prayer part of your daily routine

STEP 3
Read the Bible

STEP 4
Use the power of love

STEP 5
Become a servant of others

STEP 6
Tithe

STEP 7
Attend church regularly

KEY #1: SPIRITUALITY

Spirituality means different things to different people. For me, it means doing my best to emulate the teachings of Jesus. I am a Christian. I know non-Christians may have a different faith that is just as strong and just as valid. Some people may not conceptualize a personal God, yet hold a sense of godliness and sacredness in their everyday lives.

Please understand that when I talk about my spiritual beliefs, I am in no way trying to claim religious superiority or exclusivity. I believe that God—however or whatever you imagine God to be—works in our lives for good. And I believe God can have a profound effect on our health.

I've been in the natural health business for the past 40 years. I've spoken with thousands of people about their experiences with conventional and non-conventional therapies, with mainstream physicians and alternative practitioners, with prescription medicines and natural supplements.

I've reached the conclusion that the most powerful medicine of all may have nothing to do with drugs, surgery, or other medical "magic bullets." I have seen for myself that the human spirit is phenomenally therapeutic and can create miracles when science falls short.

STEP 1. *Realize the power of prayer*

Prayer is especially good medicine. Consider a very well-known study by cardiologist Randolph Byrd. Over a period of ten months, Dr. Byrd investigated almost 400 patients in the coronary care unit at San Francisco's General Hospital. In this randomized, double-blind study, one group of patients was prayed for by home prayer groups, while the other group was not. The people who prayed were given a brief description of each patient's ailment. Each patient in the prayed-for group had between five and seven people praying for him or her. Neither the patients, nor the doctors, nor the nurses knew who was in which group.

After 10 months, Byrd found the following differences between the two groups:

- The prayed-for patients were five times less likely to need antibiotic medication.
- The prayed-for patients were three times less likely to have their lungs fill with fluid (pulmonary edema).
- None of the prayed-for patients needed to be on mechanical ventilators. In contrast, 12 of the unprayed for patients needed help breathing.
- Fewer of the prayed-for group died.

Larry Dossey, M.D., co-chairman of the National Institutes of Health's Office of Alternative Medicine and author of *Healing Words,* said, "The evidence is simply overwhelming that prayer functions at a distance to change physical processes in a variety of organisms, from bacteria to humans" (as quoted in *"Why Prayer is Great Medicine"* by Mary Ellen Hettinger, published in *Your Health*).

If praying is good for others, can we do it for ourselves? Absolutely. Herbert Benson, M.D., founding president of the Mind/Body Medical Institute, in Boston, Massachusetts, studied the physiological changes that prayer could set into motion. He found that patients who prayed and/or meditated could elicit a relaxation response. This response includes a decrease in heart rate, breathing rate, muscle tension, and sometimes even blood pressure.

What are the medical implications? This relaxation response could have a beneficial impact on cases of hypertension, muscle tension pain, headaches, infertility, insomnia, psychological distress, cardiac arrhythmias, premenstrual syndrome, and symptoms of cancer and AIDS.

You may be thinking God has less to do with this effect than we do. You may believe the healing comes from within ourselves, not from "up above." But I feel that *within us* is exactly where God resides, and that when we pray and meditate, we unleash God's power.

Scientists are just beginning to look into the healing potential of prayer. Fortunately, we don't have to wait for controlled studies, published reports, or FDA approval to use prayer in our everyday lives. Prayer is absolutely safe and is available to each of us, whenever we wish to make use of it. Prayer costs nothing, hurts nothing, and works on many levels. It fits perfectly into any treatment plan. No matter what your particular faith, prayer can lead you to greater health—of body, mind, and soul.

STEP 2. *Make prayer part of your daily routine*

Prayer, to me, means communion with God. While formal verbal prayers are nice, I prefer to pray in silence. Rather than recite a hundred Hail Mary's, I place myself in a silent state, get in touch with my inner being, and speak to God.

I ask God to help me or whomever I am praying for. The Bible says, "You have not because you ask not...Ask and you will receive."

Between the asking and the receiving is a period of waiting—time in which, I believe, God tests our faith and trust. God has a season for all things, and God can be trusted to act in the right time. Once we ask, then we have to put away all cares and all worries and just know that it has been done.

It is also important to ask with gratitude. You never ask anyone for something without saying thank you. So when you pray, do so with gratitude to God for answering your prayer.

Set aside at least 20 to 30 minutes a day for prayer. That 20 to 30 minutes a day not only will give you the opportunity to communicate with your Creator and with yourself, but also you will find that in those minutes you'll discover new ideas, new things you never thought about, and answers to problems. They'll start coming to you because you have allowed yourself this quiet time. When we quiet ourselves, we open up the communication lines to our inner self and God. We aren't asking questions anymore, we aren't trying to think of things, we are just letting ourselves become open for information. A conversation should be two-way; we aren't just asking from God, we are also receiving. Prayer is a time when you are leaving your mind wide open.

STEP 3. *Read the Bible*

Because I am a Christian, my holy text is the Bible, but your holy guidance may take another form. I write from my own perspective, because I think reviewing and reflecting upon holy works is a universal truth. I try to read something from the Bible daily. I know this has had a powerful influence in my life. God is my Creator. He put me on this earth, and I don't think God would put me here without giving me some instructions. When we buy an appliance, we get a manual that teaches us how to use the appliance. When God put us on this earth, I believe He gave us a manual as well—the Bible. It holds all the instructions of good living: how to sow and reap, how to tithe, how to be respectful of one another, how to be a good steward, and how to be a servant, because the servant is the one who is exalted. The Bible provides the guidelines for being a good Christian. To me, being a Christian doesn't just mean what ideas I believe in. It describes the way I try to treat my family, my friends, and my employees. It's the way I try to do business. It's the way I try to live my life. I don't always succeed, but I keep striving toward these Christian standards.

The Bible gives us so many examples which clearly teach us how to live with spirituality. I have a rather broad definition of spirituality. To me it means expressing everything good that we have in our being—faith, love, hope, honor, integrity, etc. I believe that spirituality is God working through me. Spirituality is all that God brings within me, and the Bible is my guide for accessing God within me.

One of the passages in the Bible that has helped me immensely is from Proverbs 3:5-6, "Trust in the Lord with all your heart and lean not on your own understanding; in all your ways acknowledge Him, and He will make your path straight."

Sometimes things happen in our lives, and we don't understand why they happen. The Bible says that "All things happen for good to those who love the Lord." I really believe this. And, when it says "all things," it means not just some things or good things, it really means all things.

When things happen which seem to be disastrous or extremely challenging, I know that if I trust the Lord with all my heart, and I do not rely on my own understanding of the situation, God will work it out for me. I can trust the Lord and rely on Him. I do not have to worry because all things happen for good to those who love the Lord. It gives me tremendous peace of mind to know that God is taking care of me. He has seen fit to put me on this earth and get me through the world better than I can with my own understanding and efforts at trying to analyze the situation. I know God will work it out. All I need to do is trust God with all my heart and keep working in health, happiness, and faith.

STEP 4. *Use the power of love*

Expressing love is the most important factor in expressing spirituality. The Bible says in First Corinthians Chapter 13, "If I have the gift of prophecy and can fathom all mysteries and all knowledge, and if I have a faith that can move mountains, but have not love, I am nothing. If I give all I possess to the poor and surrender my body to the flames, but have not love, I gain nothing. Love is patient, love is kind. It does not envy, it does not boast, it is not proud. It is not rude, it is not self-seeking, it is not easily angered, it keeps no record of wrongs. Love does not delight in evil but rejoices with the truth. It always protects, always trusts, always hopes, always perseveres. Love never fails."

We all need to have love in our lives. Love is the most important factor between family members, friends, business associates, customers—everyone. We are all God's children. We are all human beings. We need to learn to love each other.

When we love another human being unconditionally, something wonderful happens—we get love back. One of the key principles of life is that whatever you sow, so shall you reap, but multiplied a hundred times. When you plant a tomato seed, you get a bush of tomatoes—a tomato plant that has dozens of tomatoes on it, each of which has dozens of seeds. The law of nature always gives back more than it receives. And really, it is the same for human beings. If we feel that we are lacking, it is only because we are not giving that thing which we are lacking. We all need and want love, but in order to receive love we must first give.

The principle of reaping what you sow (or of karma) applies to anything that we want. It does require faith and trust. A farmer will not go out and dig up the seed to see if it is growing. The same is true in the human process. If you disturb the process, or worry, you block the vital energy that is creating what you desire, and you have to start all over again. The farmer doesn't go into his house and sit in a rocking chair and stare out the window at the soil and worry because he hasn't seen anything happen yet. He goes about his business. He comes back one day, and suddenly, the seeds are all up. And he has hundreds and hundreds more seeds than he planted. And that's the way life is. Life works on exactly the same principles. To make a better life for ourselves and a better world, all we need to do is plant more seeds of love in the hearts of all with whom we come into contact.

Before we can love others, we must first learn to love and accept ourselves. This is a tough challenge for most people because we fail to realize that we are a part of God. If we can accept ourselves, it is much easier to accept others because, as we look at ourselves, we are looking at everyone else. Often when people do not accept others or belittle them, it is because they are trying to raise themselves up to a superior level by using others as a stepping stone. As these people with low levels of self-love and acceptance tear down others, they feel they are building themselves up. In actuality, however, they are undermining their own self-esteem and self-acceptance.

When a person criticizes or judges other people harshly, such thoughts and feelings are really tearing down his or her own health.

To paraphrase St. Matthew Chapter 7, we should not judge others. Instead of looking for the faults in other people, we should examine our own and cast them out. Our focus should be on bringing good from ourselves and others.

Through self-acceptance and self-love, we become more accepting and loving of others. Expressing spirituality to others means looking past or through human frailties and imperfections and seeing that inside each person is a spirit that is perfect and godlike. Sometimes it may be hard to look through superficial human qualities, but, for your health and that of others, try to see the true spiritual beings within rather than focus on the shortcomings of human behavior.

In Chapter 3, Key #3—*Positive Relationships*, we will discuss further the importance of love in raising human health.

The Bible clearly shows us that the servant will be the greatest among us. I think when we humble ourselves and serve others, that is where we begin our greatest reward. And we are the ones who actually receive. One of my favorite inspirational teachers, Zig Ziglar, author of *See You at the Top* and *Top Performance,* has a very powerful philosophy. Zig teaches that we can have everything we want in life if we simply help enough people get what they want. Basically, what Zig is reinforcing is the principle of being a servant of others.

I have incorporated the principle of servitude and Zig's philosophy not only in my personal life, but also in the core philosophy in my business life. The principle works. My goal is not to sell products. My goal is not to make money. Instead, my goal is to help people. That is why I employ people who believe in helping others get what they want. If people do not get what they want from one of our products, we offer a complete, unconditional, money-back guarantee. We also do our best to educate and teach people the value of good nutrition and good health. We are not concerned about the rewards for our service; we have trust and faith in God that if we follow the guidelines He has laid down for us, we will be rewarded.

In my personal life, I have found that when I help others, it makes me feel better about myself. Think about a time in your life when you helped a friend or, better yet, a stranger. How did it make you feel when you gave of yourself freely? When I have asked people the question, "Can you describe a time in your life when you felt the best about yourself?" Invariably, they will describe a time when they gave of themselves to help (serve) another human being. It is a tremendous feeling. Somehow, through a mechanism which I don't quite understand, we just tend to feel fantastic. Maybe this feeling is what God meant when He said that the servant would be the greatest of all and would be exalted.

STEP 6. *Tithe*

Tithing is probably one of the most misunderstood and most overlooked principles of life. Tithing, according to the Bible, is giving 10% of our income to God's work. Where we tithe can be an individual choice, but our tithes should really go directly to God's work, so we must choose carefully. Tithes should probably go where we get most of our spiritual support, such as our church. We can also tithe directly to the poor. The Bible says in Psalms 41:1-3, "God blesses those who are kind to the poor. He helps them out of their troubles. He protects them and keeps them alive; He publicly honors them and destroys the power of their enemies. He nurses them when they are sick, and soothes their pains and worries." Search out and determine a beneficiary for your tithe. I believe that if everybody who reads this book would tithe, their lives would be greatly enhanced. It is unbelievable what tithing can do. I have had the privilege of talking to some people who are now tithing 90% of their income, because the remaining 5% to 10% of their income is as much as most people wish they could make in a lifetime.

The only place in the Bible where God says, "Test Me, and see if I am not telling you the truth," is in Malachi Chapter 3. It reads:

> "Return to me, and I will return to you," says the Lord Almighty.
> But you ask, "How are we to return?"
> "Will a man rob God? Yet you rob me."
> But you ask, "How do we rob you?"
> "In tithes and offerings. You are under a curse—the whole nation of you—because you are robbing me. Bring the whole tithe into the store house, that there may be food in my house. Test me in this," says the Lord Almighty, "and see if I will not throw open the floodgates of heaven and pour out so much blessings that you will not have enough room for it."

I believe in the power of these words and the power of tithing. I have used tithing throughout my life. My company tithes and my family tithes, because tithing is a principle that works. I believe that if somebody wants to be healthy and successful, without any other beliefs attached, they must tithe. Tithe because God will bless you. How can you pass up this opportunity?

Step 7. *Attend church regularly*

The last step in achieving spirituality is attending church or another house of worship aligned with your beliefs. While some may consider this step the sole factor in defining a person's spirituality, I do not use it as a yardstick to measure a person's spirituality. And yet, I consider it important.

A church brings people together in a very special way. It allows people to express their spirituality, pray together, and extend love to one another. And, according to many studies, people who attend church regularly have better health.

In a recent survey of 1,473 people, a research team led by Purdue University psychologist Kenneth Ferraro found that only 59 who went to church reported ill health compared to 133 who did not. Also, 530 of the "weekly attenders" reported excellent health, compared to only 383 of the "never attenders." For the study, Dr. Ferraro looked at three aspects: frequency of attendance at church or synagogue; the experiential aspect, or sense of feeling close to God; and the specific creed or beliefs. Of these three factors, only active participation was found to make a big difference, with higher participation linked to better health. The big question is why? The researchers offered four possible explanations:

1. People who attend church regularly tend to avoid health-destructive behaviors such as smoking and using drugs or alcohol.
2. Religious activity provides a social network for coping and support that is quite different from our secular network.
3. Faith provides a special meaning and value system to help us make sense of the world and our lives.
4. Religious practice helps us cope with physical suffering and gives us hope.

I believe one of the big reasons church-going people are healthier is that they are regularly reminded of important values. Rather than material possessions, religion values human traits we all can admire: honesty, compassion, loyalty, friendship, fellowship, and love.

Chapter Two

Key #2—Positive Attitude

Step 1
Become an optimist

Step 2
Practice positive self-talk

Step 3
Ask better questions

Step 4
Employ positive affirmations

Step 5
Set positive goals

Step 6
Use positive visualization

Step 7
Read or listen to positive messages

KEY #2—POSITIVE ATTITUDE

More and more evidence clearly demonstrates that what we think and feel has a tremendous effect on the way our body functions. The most important factor in maintaining or attaining health is a consistent "positive mental attitude." Researchers in the medical and psychological fields are demonstrating that our level of optimism is a major determining factor in our level of wellness.

The steps described in this chapter are necessary not only for achieving vibrant health, but also for achieving a life full of passion, happiness, joy, and fun. View your attitude as an entity like the human body. It needs nourishment, care, and conditioning. For most people, a positive attitude doesn't happen all at once. It happens by degrees, subtle changes accumulating one by one. Would you be in good physical condition if you exercised only once? No. It takes conditioning. The same is true for your attitude.

Life is full of events beyond our control. However, while we do not have any control over these events, we do have control over our response to them. Our attitude determines how we view and respond to the challenges of life. You will be much happier, healthier, and more successful if you can adopt a positive mental attitude rather than a pessimistic view.

STEP 1. *Become an optimist*

The first step in developing a positive mental attitude is to become an optimist. This shouldn't be too hard. According to Martin Seligman, Ph.D., author of *Learned Optimism* and one of the world's leading authorities on optimism, we are, by nature, optimists. Optimism is a necessary step towards achieving health as well as our goals in life. Research is revealing that optimism not only prevents disease, but also is a vital ally in the healing process. Conversely, a pessimistic attitude can seriously erode our health.

Several research studies indicate that chronically angry, suspicious, and mistrustful people are twice as likely to have coronary artery blockages. And during periods of grief, the T cells—important white blood cells which fight against infection and cancer—do not multiply as quickly.

What distinguishes an optimist from a pessimist is the way that each explains both good and bad events. Dr. Seligman has developed a simple test to determine your level of optimism. Try his test and evaluate your outlook.

Are you an optimist?

To determine whether you are an optimist, answer the following questions. Take as much time as you need. There are no right or wrong answers. It is important that you take the test before you read the interpretation. Read the description of each situation and vividly imagine it happening to you. Choose the response that most applies to you by circling either A or B. Ignore the letter and number codes for now; they will be explained later.

Test your optimism

1. The project you are in charge of is a great success.

	PsG
A. *I kept a close watch over everyone's work.*	1
B. *Everyone devoted a lot of time and energy to it.*	0

2. You and your spouse (boyfriend/girlfriend) make up after a fight.

	PmG
A. *I forgave him/her.*	0
B. *I'm usually forgiving.*	1

3. You get lost driving to a friend's house.

	PsB
A. *I missed a turn.*	1
B. *My friend gave me bad directions.*	0

4. Your spouse (boyfriend/girlfriend) surprises you with a gift.

	PsG
A. *He/she just got a raise at work.*	0
B. *I took him/her out to a special dinner the night before.*	1

5. You forgot your spouse's (boyfriend's/girlfriend's) birthday.

	PmB
A. *I'm not good at remembering birthdays.*	1
B. *I was preoccupied with other things.*	0

6. You get a flower from a secret admirer.

	PvG
A. *I am attractive to him/her.*	0
B. *I am a popular person.*	1

7. You run for a community office position and you win.

	PvG
A. *I devote a lot of time and energy to campaigning.*	0
B. *I work very hard at everything I do.*	1

8. You miss an important engagement.

	PvB
A. *Sometimes my memory fails me.*	1
B. *I sometimes forget to check my appointment book.*	0

9. You run for a community office position and you lose.

	PsB
A. *I didn't campaign hard enough.*	1
B. *The person who won knew more people.*	0

10. You host a successful dinner.

	PmG
A. *I was particularly charming that night.*	0
B. *I am a good host.*	1

11. You stop a crime by calling the police.

	PsG
A. *A strange noise caught my attention.*	0
B. *I was alert that day.*	1

12. You were extremely healthy all year.

	PsG
A. *Few people around me were sick, so I wasn't exposed.*	0
B. *I made sure I ate well and got enough rest.*	1

13. You owe the library ten dollars for an overdue book.

	PmB
A. *When I am really involved in what I am reading, I often forget when it's due.*	1
B. *I was so involved in writing the report that I forgot to return the book.*	0

14. Your stocks make you a lot of money.

	PmG
A. *My broker decided to take on something new.*	0
B. *My broker is a top-notch investor.*	1

15. You win an athletic contest.

	PmG
A. *I was feeling unbeatable.*	0
B. *I train hard.*	1

16. You fail an important examination.

                                                            PvB

A. I wasn't as smart as the other people taking the exam.   1

B. I didn't prepare for it well.   0

17. You prepared a special meal for a friend and he/she barely touched the food.

      PvB

A. I wasn't a good cook.   1

B. I made the meal in a rush.   0

18. You lose a sporting event for which you have been training for a long time.

      PvB

A. I'm not very athletic.   1

B. I'm not good at that sport.   0

19. Your car runs out of gas on a dark street late at night.

      PsB

A. I didn't check to see how much gas was in the tank.   1

B. The gas gauge was broken.   0

20. You lose your temper with a friend.

      PmB

A. He/she is always nagging me.   1

B. He/she was in a hostile mood.   0

21. You are penalized for not returning your income-tax forms on time.

      PmB

A. I always put off doing my taxes.   1

B. I was lazy about getting my taxes done this year.   0

22. You ask a person out on a date and he/she says no.

      PvB

A. I was a wreck that day.   1

B. I got tongue-tied when I asked him/her on the date.   0

23. A game-show host picks you out of the audience to participate in the show.

      PsG

A. I was sitting in the right seat.   0

B. I looked the most enthusiastic.   1

24. You are frequently asked to dance at a party.

      PmG

A. I am outgoing at parties.   1

B. I was in perfect form that night.   0

25. You buy your spouse (boyfriend/girlfriend) a gift and he/she doesn't like it.

	PsB
A. *I don't put enough thought into things like that.*	1
B. *He/she has very picky tastes.*	0

26. You do exceptionally well in a job interview.

	PmG
A. *I felt extremely confident during the interview.*	0
B. *I interview well.*	1

27. You tell a joke and everyone laughs.

	PsG
A. *The joke was funny.*	0
B. *My timing was perfect.*	1

28. Your boss gives you too little time in which to finish a project, but you get it finished anyway.

	PvG
A. *I am good at my job.*	0
B. *I am an efficient person.*	1

29. You've been feeling run-down lately.

	PmB
A. *I never get a chance to relax.*	1
B. *I was exceptionally busy this week.*	0

30. You ask someone to dance and he/she says no.

	PsB
A. *I am not a good enough dancer.*	1
B. *He/she doesn't like to dance.*	0

31. You save a person from choking to death.

	PvG
A. *I know a technique to stop someone from choking.*	0
B. *I know what to do in crisis situations.*	1

32. Your romantic partner wants to cool things off for a while.

	PvB
A. *I'm too self-centered.*	1
B. *I don't spend enough time with him/her.*	0

33. A friend says something that hurts your feelings.

	PmB
A. *She always blurts things out without thinking of others.*	1
B. *My friend was in a bad mood and took it out on me.*	0

34. Your employer comes to you for advice.

	PvG
A. *I am an expert in the area about which I was asked.*	0
B. *I'm good at giving useful advice.*	1

35. A friend thanks you for helping him/her get through a bad time.

	PvG
A. *I enjoy helping him/her through tough times.*	0
B. *I care about people.*	1

36. You have a wonderful time at a party.

	PsG
A. *Everyone was friendly.*	0
B. *I was friendly.*	1

37. Your doctor tells you that you are in good physical shape.

	PvG
A. *I make sure I exercise frequently.*	0
B. *I am very health-conscious.*	1

38. Your spouse (boyfriend/girlfriend) takes you away for a romantic weekend.

	PmG
A. *He/she needed to get away for a few days.*	0
B. *He/she likes to explore new areas.*	1

39. Your doctor tells you that you eat too much sugar.

	PsB
A. *I don't pay much attention to my diet.*	1
B. *You can't avoid sugar, it's in everything.*	0

40. You are asked to head an important project.

	PmG
A. *I just successfully completed a similar project.*	0
B. *I am a good supervisor.*	1

41. You and your spouse (boyfriend/girlfriend) have been fighting a great deal.

	PsB
A. *I have been feeling cranky and pressured lately.*	1
B. *He/she has been hostile lately.*	0

42. You fall down a great deal while skiing.

	PmB
A. *Skiing is difficult.*	1
B. *The trails were icy.*	0

43. You win a prestigious award.

	PvG
A. I solved an important problem.	0
B. I was the best employee.	1

44. Your stocks are at an all-time low.

	PvB
A. I didn't know much about the business climate at the time.	1
B. I made a poor choice of stocks.	0

45. You win the lottery.

	PsG
A. It was pure chance.	0
B. I picked the right numbers.	1

46. You gain weight over the holidays and you can't lose it.

	PmB
A. Diets don't work in the long run.	1
B. The diet I tried didn't work.	0

47. You are in the hospital and few people come to visit.

	PsB
A. I'm irritable when I am sick.	1
B. My friends are negligent about things like that.	0

48. They won't honor your credit card at a store.

	PvB
A. I sometimes overestimate how much money I have.	1
B. I sometimes forget to pay my credit card bill.	0

Scoring Key

PmB _____   PmG _____

PvB _____   PvG _____

HoB _____

PsB _____   PsG _____

Total B _____   Total G _____

G-B _____

Interpreting your test

The test results will give you a clue as to your explanatory style. In other words, the results will tell you how you explain things to yourself. It will show you your habitual way of thinking. Again, remember, there are no right or wrong answers.

Your explanatory style is composed of three crucial dimensions: permanence, pervasiveness, and personalization. Each dimension, plus a couple of others, will be scored from your test.

Permanence

When pessimists are faced with challenges or bad events, they view these events as being permanent. In contrast, people who are optimists tend to view the challenges or bad events as temporary. Here are some statements that reflect some subtle differences

Pessimistic (Permanent)	Optimistic (Temporary)
"My boss is always a jerk."	"My boss is in a bad mood today."
"You never listen."	"You are not listening."
"I'm an unlucky person."	"This event was unfortunate."

To determine how you view bad events, look at the eight items coded PmB (for Permanent Bad): 5, 13, 20, 21, 29, 33, 42, and 46. Each one followed by a 0 is optimistic, while each one followed by a 1 is pessimistic. Total the numbers at the right-hand margin of the questions coded PmB and write the total on the PmB line on the scoring key.

If you totaled 0 or 1, you are very optimistic in this dimension; 2 or 3 is a moderately optimistic score; 4 is average; 5 or 6 is pessimistic; a 7 or 8 is extremely pessimistic.

Now let's take a look at the difference in explanatory style between pessimists and optimists when a positive event occurs in their lives. It's just the opposite of what happened with a bad event. Pessimists view positive events as temporary while optimists view them as permanent. Here again are some subtle differences in how pessimists and optimists might communicate their good fortune:

Pessimistic (Temporary)	Optimistic (Permanent)
"I'm lucky for once."	"I'm such a lucky person."
"My opponent was off today."	"I am getting better every day."
"I tried hard today."	"I always give my best."

Now total all the questions coded PmG (for Permanent Good): 2, 10, 14, 15, 24, 26, 38, and 40. Write the total on the line in the scoring key marked PmG.

If you totaled 7 or 8, you are very optimistic in this dimension; 6 is a moderately optimistic score; 4 or 5 is average; 3 is pessimistic; a 0, 1 or 2 is extremely pessimistic.

Are you starting to see a pattern? If you are scoring as a pessimist, you may want to learn how to be more optimistic. Your anxiety may be due to your belief that bad things are always going to happen, while good things are only a fluke.

Pervasiveness

Pervasiveness is the tendency to describe things in universals (everyone, always, never, etc.) versus specifics (a specific individual, a specific time, etc.). Pessimists tend to describe things in universals while optimists describe things in specifics.

Pessimist (Universal)	Optimist (Specific)
"All lawyers are jerks."	"My attorney was a jerk."
"He is repulsive."	"He is repulsive to me."
"Instruction manuals are worthless."	"This instruction manual is worthless."

Total your score for the questions coded PvB (for Pervasive Bad): 8, 16, 17, 18, 22, 32, 44, and 48. Write the total on the PvB line.

If you totaled 0 or 1, you are very optimistic in this dimension; 2 or 3 is a moderately optimistic score; 4 is average; 5 or 6 is pessimistic; a 7 or 8 is extremely pessimistic.

Now let's look at the level of pervasiveness of good events. Optimists tend to view good events as universal, while pessimists view them as specific. Again, it's just the opposite of how each views a bad event.

Total your score for the questions coded PvG (for Pervasive Good): 6, 7, 28, 31, 34, 35, 37, and 43. Write the total on the line labeled PvG.

If you totaled 7 or 8, you are very optimistic in this dimension; 6 is a moderately optimistic score; 4 or 5 is average; 3 is pessimistic; a 0, 1 or 2 is extremely pessimistic.

Hope

Our level of hope or hopelessness is determined by our combined level of permanence and pervasiveness. Your level of hope may be the most significant score for this test. Take your PvB and add it to your PmB score. This is your hope score.

If it is 0, 1, or 2, you are extraordinarily hopeful; 3, 4, 5, or 6 is a moderately hopeful score; 7 or 8 is average; 9, 10, or 11 is moderately hopeless; and 12, 13, 14, 15, or 16 is severely hopeless.

People who make permanent and universal explanations for their troubles tend to suffer from stress, anxiety, and depression. When things go bad, they collapse. According to Dr. Seligman, no other score is as important as your hope score.

Personalization

The final aspect of explanatory style is personalization. When bad things happen, we can either assume all the blame ourselves (internalize) and lower our self-esteem as a consequence, or we can put some of the blame on things beyond our control (externalize). Although it may not be right to deny any personal responsibility, people who tend to externalize some of the blame for bad events have higher self-esteem and are more optimistic.

Total your score for the questions coded PsB (for Personalization Bad): 3, 9, 19, 25, 30, 39, 41, and 47. Write the total on the PsB line. A score of 0 or 1 indicates very high self-esteem and optimism; 2 or 3 indicates moderate self-esteem; 4 is average; 5 or 6 indicates moderately low self-esteem; and 7 or 8 indicates very low self-esteem.

Now let's take a look at personalization and good events. Again, just the exact opposite interpretation occurs compared to bad events. When good things happen, the person with high self-esteem internalizes while the person with low self-esteem externalizes.

Total your score for the questions coded PsG (for Personalization Good): 1, 4, 11, 12, 23, 27, 36, and 45. Write your total on the line marked PsG on the scoring key.

If you totaled 7 or 8, you are very optimistic in this dimension; 6 is a moderately optimistic score; 4 or 5 is average; 3 is pessimistic; a 0, 1 or 2 is extremely pessimistic.

Your overall scores

To compute your overall scores, first add the three Bs (PmB + PvB + PsB). This is your B (bad event) score. Do the same for all of the Gs (PmG

+ PvG + PsG). This is your G (good event) score. Subtract B from G; this is your overall score.

If your B score is from 3 to 6, you are marvelously optimistic when bad events occur; 10 or 11 is average; 12 to 14 is pessimistic; anything above 14 is extremely pessimistic.

If your G score is 19 or above, you are extremely optimistic in your thoughts about good events; 14 to 16 is average; 11 to 13 indicates pessimism; and a score of 10 or less indicates great pessimism.

If your overall score (G minus B) is above 8, you are very optimistic across the board; if it's from 6 to 8 you are moderately optimistic; 3 to 5 is average; 1 or 2 is pessimistic; and a score of zero or below is very pessimistic.

Optimism and health

Optimists have been shown to possess greater health. Consider the findings of researcher Christopher Peterson, Ph.D., professor of psychology at the University of Michigan. He and his colleagues analyzed data from a 35-year research project known as the Harvard Study of Adult Development. The 268 men in the study were drawn from the Harvard classes of 1942 and 1944. They were chosen on the basis of their academic success, sound physical and psychological health, and high level of independence and accomplishment as determined by college deans.

Test subjects' optimism scores were compared with their health ratings as determined by doctors. They underwent physical exams at age 25 and every five years afterward. It's no surprise that those who scored higher for optimism remained healthier later in life than the men who were more pessimistic.

Naturally, optimistic people are more inclined to look after their own health. They are more likely to work out, eat a balanced diet, and get regular medical checkups. Optimists respond to illness actively, consulting their doctor promptly and following a responsible treatment plan.

Learning optimism

It is important to learn how to be optimistic if you are a pessimist. Why? Again, studies have shown that optimists are healthier, happier, and enjoy life at a much higher level than pessimists. Learning to be optimistic means that you need to get in the habit of thinking with a positive attitude. If you are pessimistic, it is only because you habitually think in a negative framework.

Is it possible to learn optimism? More psychologists are saying yes. Cognitive therapy, originally developed by psychiatrist Aaron T. Beck and psychologist Albert Ellis, is based on the premise that our thoughts control our feelings. In other words, if we can adopt more positive habits of thought, we can make ourselves feel better.

The Complete Guide to Your Emotions & Your Health, by Emrika Padus and the editors of *Prevention* magazine, explains that negative thinking is a learned response. Six common pessimistic distortions are exaggerating, ignoring the positive, personalizing, either/or thinking, over-generalizing, and jumping to conclusions. Gary Emery, Ph.D., author of *A New Beginning*, writes, "The chief characteristic of negative thoughts is that they're generally wrong."

To "reprogram" your thinking, *The Complete Guide* suggests that you become aware of the unfocused negative thoughts that leap into your mind uninvited. Write them down. Then respond to them with more realistic, constructive, and adaptive thinking.

Another book, *Feeling Good*, by David Burns, offers the following suggestions for becoming more optimistic:

Choose an area of your life in which you want to begin thinking and acting more optimistically.

- Become aware of your thoughts and beliefs in this area.
- Ask yourself how realistic these beliefs are.
- Set modest and immediate goals for changing your habits of thinking.
- As you make those changes successfully, reward yourself.
- Seek out the company of optimistic people.
- Be playful about your venture into optimism.
- Remember that optimism is healthy, in part, because it leads to action.
- Ask your friends and family members to help you.
- Make some positive changes in your lifestyle.
- Be flexible. Use these suggestions in whatever way seems best to you.
- Don't let setbacks or delays discourage you.

Cognitive thinking is a skill-building process. With time, effort, and commitment, anyone can replace the habit of negative thinking with a new habit of more constructive, positive thinking. And that's a vital step toward better health.

STEP 2. *Practice positive self-talk*

To be truly healthy, we must have positive self-talk. By self-talk, I am referring to the type of language used by your brain. Self-talk is a powerful tool in creating a positive attitude.

Self-talk plugs directly into our subconscious, which either tells us how we are going to feel or starts the process of creating a "self-fulfilling prophecy." For example, how do you usually respond when somebody says, "How are you?" I believe that your routine answer to this question goes a long way in determining your dominant emotional and physical state. If your answer is "not too bad," then that becomes your dominant state. If your answer is "O.K.," then that becomes your dominant state.

When people ask me how I am, I always say something like "super," "great," "fantastic," "phenomenal," or, on occasion, "ecstatic." Even though I may not feel great that day, in time, if I continue to say how I want to feel, then that will become my dominant state. I know this may sound kind of strange, but all I can say is try it for yourself. It's fun to watch how people respond. Usually they will say, "Wow, what is going on in your life that is so fantastic?" Your response to this question is to focus on all of the positive things in your life which, in turn, increases your positive mental attitude and attracts even more things to be thankful for.

Some people might have a hard time believing in the power of positive self-talk, but if they take the opportunity to use it, I know it can dramatically improve the quality of their life. Two powerful tools for creating positive self-talk are questions and affirmations (discussed next).

STEP 3. *Ask better questions*

One of the most powerful tools I have found for improving the quality of my self-talk and the quality of my life is a series of questions originally given to me by Anthony Robbins, author of the bestsellers, *Unlimited Power* and *Awaken the Giant Within*. According to Tony, the quality of your life is equal to the quality of the questions you habitually ask yourself. Tony's statement is based on his belief that whatever question you ask your brain is the question your brain will answer.

Let's look at the following example: An individual is met with a particular challenge or problem. He or she can ask a number of questions in this situation. Questions many people ask in such circumstances include: "Why does this always happen to me?" Or, "Why am I always so stupid?" Do they get answers to these questions? Do the answers build self-esteem? Does the problem keep reappearing? What would be a higher quality question?

How about: "This is a very interesting situation. What do I need to learn from this situation so it never happens again?" Or, "What can I do to make this situation better?"

In another example, let's look at an individual who suffers from depression. What are some questions he or she might ask which may not be helping the situation? How about: "Why am I always so depressed?" "Why do things always seem to go wrong for me?" "Why am I doomed to be so unhappy?"

What are some better questions they may want to ask themselves? How about: "What do I need to do to gain more enjoyment and happiness in my life?" "What do I need to commit to in order to have more happiness and energy in my life?" After they have answered these questions, they could ask themselves this one: "If I had happiness and high energy levels right now, what would it feel like?"

You will be amazed at how powerful questions can be in your life. When the mind is searching for answers to these questions, it is reprogramming your subconscious into believing you have an abundance of energy. Unless there is a physiological reason for the chronic fatigue, it won't take long before your subconscious believes.

Regardless of the situation, asking better questions is bound to improve your attitude. If you want to have a better life, simply ask better questions. It sounds simple because it is. If you want more energy, excitement, and happiness in your life, ask yourself the following questions on a consistent basis.

The Morning Questions
1. What am I most happy about in my life right now?

    Why does that make me happy? How does that make me feel?
2. What am I most excited about in my life right now?

    Why does that make me excited? How does that make me feel?
3. What am I most grateful for in my life right now?

    Why does that make me grateful? How does that make me feel?
4. What am I enjoying most about my life right now?

    What about that do I enjoy? How does that make me feel?
5. What am I committed to in my life right now?

    Why am I committed to that? How does that make me feel?
6. Who do I love? (Starting close and moving out) Who loves me?
7. What must I do today to achieve my long-term goal?

The Evening Questions

1. What have I given today? In what ways have I been a giver today?
2. What did I learn today?
3. What did I do today to reach my long-term goal?
4. In what ways was today a perfect day?
5. Repeat morning questions.

The Problem or Challenge Questions

1. What is right/great about this problem?
2. What is not perfect yet?
3. What am I willing to do to make it the way I want it to be?
4. How can I enjoy doing the things necessary to make it the way I want it to be?

STEP 4. *Employ positive affirmations*

An affirmation is a positive statement. Affirmations can make imprints on the subconscious mind to create a healthy, positive self-image. In addition, affirmations can actually fuel the changes you desire. I use certain phrases and sentences as affirmations each day. Some of my favorites are:

- I can do all things through Christ who gives me the strength.
- I feel healthy. I feel great. I feel terrific.
- Money flows through me freely for the good of others.
- Love flows through me in avalanches of abundance.

Here are some very simple guidelines for creating your own affirmations.

1. Always phrase an affirmation in the present tense. Imagine that it has already come to pass.
2. Always phrase the affirmation as a positive statement. Avoid the words "not" or "never."
3. Do your best to totally identify with the positive feelings that are generated by the affirmation.
4. Keep the affirmation short and simple but full of feeling. Be creative.
5. Imagine yourself really experiencing what you are affirming.
6. Make the affirmation personal to you and full of meaning.

Using these guidelines and examples, write down five affirmations that apply to you. State these affirmations aloud while you are taking your shower, driving, or when you are praying.

STEP 5. *Set positive goals*

Learning to set goals in a positive way is another powerful method for building a positive attitude and raising self-esteem. Goals can be used to create a "success cycle." Achieving goals helps you feel better about yourself, and the better you feel about yourself, the more likely you will achieve your goals. Here are some guidelines to use when setting goals.

>   1. State the goal in positive terms; avoid any negative words in your goal statement. For example, it is better to say "I enjoy eating healthy, low-calorie, nutritious foods" than "I will not eat sugar, candy, ice cream, and other fattening foods." Remember, always state the goal in positive terms, and avoid any negative words in the goal statement.

>   2. Make your goal attainable and realistic. Again, you can use goals to create a success cycle and positive self-image. Little things add up to make a major difference in the way you feel about yourself.

>   3. Be specific. The more clearly your goal is defined, the more likely you are to reach it. For example, if you want to lose weight, what is the weight you desire? What body fat percentage or measurements do you desire? Clearly define just what you want to achieve.

>   4. State the goal in the present tense, not the future tense. In order to reach your goal, you have to believe you have already attained it. You must literally program yourself to achieve the goal. See and feel yourself having already achieved the goal and success will be yours. Remember, always state your goal in the present tense.

Any voyage begins with one step and is followed by many other steps. Remember to set short-term goals which can be used to help you achieve your long-term goals. Get in the habit of asking yourself the following question each morning and evening: What must I do today to achieve my long-term goal?

STEP 6. *Use positive visualization*

Positive visualization or imagery is another powerful tool for creating health, happiness, and success. I believe that we have to be able to see our lives the way we want them to be before it happens.

A number of excellent books can help inspire you with accounts of the power of positive visualization. One of the first books I read on this subject was Maxwell Maltz's now classic work, *Psycho-Cybernetics*. Another excellent book is Dr. Wayne Dyer's *You'll See It When You Believe It.*

Most of the initial research on the power of visualization focused on enhancing physical performance. For example, in *Psycho-Cybernetics*, Maltz recounts an experiment comparing the effect of visualization versus physical practice in improving basketball free throw shooting.

One group of students actually practiced shooting free throws for twenty minutes each day for twenty days and were scored on the first and last day. A second group was scored on the first and last days, but engaged in no sort of practice in between. A third group was scored on the first and last days, but spent twenty minutes on each of the intervening days visualizing shooting free throws successfully.

The results? Visualization was just as effective as actual physical practice. The first group improved 24%, the second group showed no improvement, and the third group improved 23%.

The power of positive visualization is discussed extensively in *Peak Performance* by Dr. Charles Garfield, a psychologist who has done extensive research on peak performance, both in business and athletics. While working with the NASA program, Dr. Garfield became fascinated with the power of visualization as he watched astronauts rehearse scenes over and over in their heads, so they would be prepared when they went into space. Although he had a doctorate in mathematics, he decided to go back to school and get a Ph.D. in the field of psychology. His focus was to better understand the characteristics of successful people.

One of Dr. Garfield's key findings is that almost all world-class athletes and other peak performers employ positive visualization. They see their goal, they feel it, and identify with it so strongly emotionally that they actually experience it before they do it. It all begins in the mind's eye.

You can use visualization in all areas of your life, but especially for your health. In fact, some of the most promising research on the power of visualization involves enhancing the immune system in the treatment of cancer. Much of the pioneering work in this field has been conducted at the Simonton Research Center in Dallas, Texas, under the supervision of Carl Simonton, M.D. Along with standard medical treatment, Dr. Simonton teaches patients how to imagine white blood cells as little Pac-Men digesting and destroying tumors. Dr. Simonton's techniques are described in his book, *Getting Well Again*.

Dr. Simonton and others are showing that positive visualization is proving to be very powerful medicine. For example, a study conducted at Yale University demonstrated that patients suffering from severe depression were helped considerably by simply imagining scenes in which they were praised by people they admired. Be creative and have fun with positive visualizations, and you will soon find yourself living your dreams.

To help get you started, here is an excellent visualization script excerpted from *Rituals of Healing—Using Imagery for Health and Wellness* by Jeanne Acterberg, Barbara Dossey, and Leslie Kolkmeier. Use it to promote overall healing and general well-being.

Before you begin your imagery journey, find a quiet, comfortable place, and give yourself permission to spend fifteen or twenty minutes taking care of yourself. Lie down, or sit with your back and neck completely supported. Allow your chair, or bed, or wherever you are to hold you. Let tension melt away as you bring your attention to your breath, listening to, feeling the in breath, the out breath...[Pause for one minute.] Take a mental journey now, through your body, beginning at the bottom of your feet. Move your attention slowly to the top of your head, letting go of any tightness or restriction you find. [Pause for one or two minutes, or guide yourself through your muscle groups.]

Your mind has just moved through your body, connecting with it, giving it attention, soothing the tense, tired places. Now let your mind move to a still point. Some people find this still point deep within, a place of pure peace and calm, a place of quiet knowing. Let the words "still point" fill your mind, chasing out other thoughts and concerns. Breathe yourself into this quiet place. Quietly, gently find the stillness. [Pause one minute.]

Sit comfortably, with your back straight but relaxed. Focus on your breath and inhale and exhale three times. Then, slowly, begin to inhale.

As you feel the air moving in through your nose and down the back of your throat into your lungs, hear yourself saying, way in the back of your mind..."One."...Feel the air moving back out...As the next breath begins to fill your lungs, hear yourself saying, deep inside of yourself..."Two."... Feel the air moving back out...With the next breath in, hear yourself saying, deep inside of yourself..."Three."...Feel the air moving back out...With the next breath in, hear yourself saying, deep inside of yourself..."Four."...

Feel the air moving back out…Repeat this cycle as many times as you wish, counting one to four with your breaths.

With each breath in…feel your diaphragm moving down toward your feet…and your lower abdomen beginning to expand…With each breath out…as your abdomen relaxes…feel the muscles in your neck and shoulders drifting down with gravity…and relaxing even more deeply.

Imagine your body is made of a beautiful, clear, crystalline material…Each time you breathe in, imagine your breath is a healing, colored mist…any color that comes to mind…Feel the healing mist entering your body through the top of your head and drifting slowly down inside your crystal-clear body…See and feel that mist beginning to fill you with relaxation and calm…Each breath slowly fills your crystal body with peace and healing…Continue to see yourself filling with color until your body is completely full of relaxation.

With the next breath in, say to yourself, "I am breathing…" As you breathe out, say to yourself, "warmth into my feet."…With the next breath in, say to yourself, "I am breathing…" As you breathe out, say to yourself, "warmth into my legs."…Continue in this manner, breathing warmth into all parts of your body…Gradually come back to full awareness of the room and notice your calmness and relaxation.

This relaxation technique is phenomenally effective for dealing with stress. It feels fantastic to let go of all the pressures of modern living. I use this technique often not only for visualization exercises, but also for magnifying prayer and meditation.

Realizing that our actions, feelings, and behavior are the results of our internal images gives us a powerful tool for gaining new skills, success, greater happiness, and better health.

Step 7. *Read or listen to positive messages*

Achieving a positive mental attitude is very similar to achieving a highly conditioned physical body. Just like the physical body, we must exercise and condition our attitude. All of the steps discussed in this chapter are important in this effort. The final step, reading or listening to positive messages, is one that helps me continually renew my motivation and inspiration. While driving, exercising, cooking, or doing chores around the house, I take advantage of CDs that nourish my attitude with good, positive, inspirational information. Before going to sleep, I always take a few minutes to read something that fills my mind with positive thoughts.

Here are some of the authors and books (in alphabetical order by author) that have inspired me the most. Most of these authors also have audio books available. A good resource is the Nightingale-Conant company (1-800-525-9000).

Buscaglia, Leo
Living, Loving, and Learning
Loving Each Other

Carnegie, Dale
How to Win Friends & Influence People

Covey, Stephen R.
The 7 Habits of Highly Effective People
Principle-Centered Leadership

Frankl, Victor
Man's Search for Meaning

Hill, Napoleon
Think and Grow Rich

Jampolsky, Gerald
Love is Letting Go of Fear

Mandino, Og
Mission Success
The Greatest Salesman in the World
The Greatest Success in the World

McGinnis, Alan Loy
The Friendship Factor
Bringing Out the Best in People

Peale, Norman Vincent
The Power of Positive Thinking
Bible Power for Successful Living

Robbins, Anthony
Unlimited Power
Awaken the Giant Within

Seligman, Martin
Learned Optimism
What You Can Change...and What You Can't

Waitley, Denis
The Double Win Being the Best Seeds of Greatness

Ziglar, Zig
Confession of a Happy Christian
See You at the Top
Top Performance

CHAPTER THREE

KEY #3—POSITIVE RELATIONSHIPS

STEP 1
Learn to help others

STEP 2
Develop positive qualities

STEP 3
Learn to listen

STEP 4
Find the good

STEP 5
Demonstrate love and appreciation

STEP 6
Develop intimacy

STEP 7
Recognize challenges in relationships

Key #3—Positive Relationships

Human beings need each other. We need to work with others, exchange services, share information, and provide emotional comfort. Positive human relationships sustain us and nourish us—body and soul.

Without positive human relationships, we cannot be healthy. What happens when we're cut off from others? In an experiment cited in *Bible Power for Successful Living,* by Norman Vincent Peale, a hospital staff assessed the impact of isolation on their own mascot. While I am not in favor of this kind of experimentation on a pet, the examinations were done in a painless manner, and I think the results are too important to ignore. This dog had typically been lavished with attention and affection. When staff members made a very small incision in a bone in the dog's leg, they found it in healthy, pink condition. After the first incision, the hospital staff ignored the dog for a few days. They stopped petting it or paying it any attention. The dog was miserable. They made another small incision, and found that the interior of the bone was brown and dry. Finally, the staff started to greet and pet the dog as they had done originally. When they made the third incision, once more the bone tissue looked pink and healthy.

This situation brings to mind Proverbs 17:22, "A merry heart doeth good like medicine: but a broken spirit drieth the bones."

Loneliness affects us—even on a cellular level. In fact, poor personal relationships and lack of social support can actually damage the immune system, according to *Mind/Body Medicine*, edited by Daniel Goleman, Ph.D., and Joel Gurin. Researchers who have studied diverse groups of people have found that those who are lonely—as assessed by psychological tests—are more likely to have sluggish immune systems.

There's still more evidence that loneliness can make us sick. Sociologist James House and colleagues investigated data from large, well-controlled population studies. They concluded that unsatisfactory social relationships were as important a risk factor for heart disease and premature death as smoking, high blood pressure, high blood cholesterol, obesity, and inactivity.

If loneliness leads to illness, it makes sense that love and positive human relationships are truly the road to health. In a study of almost 7,000 adults in Alameda County, California, researchers Lisa Berkman, Ph.D., and S. Leonard Syme, Ph.D., found that people with more social contacts were two to five times more likely to outlive their more isolated counterparts.

At Tel Aviv University in Israel, a five-year study of almost 10,000 men diagnosed as having a high risk of heart disease found they were almost twice as likely not to develop angina pectoris—chest pain from restriction of blood to the heart—if they felt they had loving and supportive wives. Researchers were surprised to discover that other risk factors, including hypertension and high cholesterol, were also significantly reduced if a husband believed he had his wife's love and support.

Dr. Ken Pelletier, of the University of California, San Francisco, School of Medicine, and author of *Mind as Healer, Mind as Slayer* says, "Community support groups and close personal relationships have been linked to better health and lower absenteeism, lower incidence of cancer and heart disease, and reduced hospital stays." In one study cited by Dr. Pelletier, researchers divided 1,337 medical students into two groups: one made up of students who were not close to their parents and were dissatisfied with their personal relationships, and one that was psychologically healthier. The first group was found to have a three to four times higher risk of cancer later in life than the healthier students.

Dr. Pelletier pointed out that people who feel they don't have enough social support are more susceptible to arthritis, tuberculosis, high blood pressure, and heart disease. He stated, "There is a link between disease and depression, loneliness, and hopelessness that's been shown in research."

A community that demonstrated the health benefits of the ties that bind was Roseto, Pennsylvania. A study published in the *American Journal of Public Health* showed that in this closely knit community of Italian-Americans, despite their high-fat diet, heart disease rates were significantly lower than those in neighboring towns and the rest of the United States. However, when younger members moved away from the community, their rate of heart disease climbed substantially and began to equal national norms.

This appears to be true all over the world. People in Japan are known for their strong attachment to community. They also enjoy the longest life expectancy in the world. And people in less developed societies who are close to their neighbors have lower blood pressure and fewer symptoms of heart problems than individuals in more advanced societies, who are more distant from their neighbors. Is this coincidence? I don't think so.

Do the negative feelings themselves cause illness, or are unhappy people less inclined to take good care of themselves? Perhaps the distinction is immaterial. If we can take control of our thoughts and feelings, perhaps we can learn to take greater control of our health.

STEP 1. *Learn to help others*

Altruism is defined as unselfish concern for the welfare of others. Although its focus is on others, altruistic love does serve the self indirectly by promoting health.

Allan Luks, former executive director of the Institute for the Advancement of Health, distributed questionnaires to 3,000 volunteers. He found that "People who help others frequently report better health than people who don't." He also found that over 90% of respondents reported positive physical sensations linked to helping others: exhilaration, strength, and tranquility. Kathy Keeton, author of *Longevity*, writes, "It's becoming increasingly clear that a helpful, caring attitude toward others may be a ticket not only to a happier and more productive life, but to a longer life as well."

There's a universal truth that too few people in this world really believe in: By helping others, we help ourselves. In Chapter 1, Step 5, I urged you to begin as a servant of others. Adopting this attitude will produce dramatic changes in the quality of your life, especially in your personal relationships.

Here is a story from Zig Ziglar's *See You at the Top* that really demonstrates how important it is for us to help one another.

"A man was given a tour of both Heaven and Hell, so he could intelligently select his final destination. The Devil was given first chance, so he started the 'prospect' with a tour of Hell. The first glance was a surprising one because all occupants were seated at a banquet table loaded with every food imaginable, including meat from every corner of the globe, fruits and vegetables and every delicacy known to man. With justification, the Devil pointed out that no one could ask for more.

"However, when the man looked carefully at the people he did not find a single smile. He heard no music nor did he see any indication of the gaiety generally associated with such a feast. The people at the table looked dull and listless and were literally skin and bones. The tourist noticed that each person had a fork strapped to the left arm and a knife strapped to the right arm. Each had a four-foot handle which made it impossible to eat. So, with food of every kind at their fingertips, they were starving.

"Next stop was Heaven, where the tourist saw a scene identical in every respect—same foods, same knives and forks with those four-foot handles. However, the inhabitants of Heaven were laughing, singing, and having a great time. They were well-fed and in excellent health. The tourist was puzzled for a moment. He wondered how conditions could be so similar and yet produce such different results. The people in Hell were starving and miserable, while the people in Heaven were well-fed and happy. Then, he saw the reason. Each person in Hell had been trying to feed himself. A knife and fork with a four-foot handle made this impossible. Each person in Heaven was feeding the one across the table from him and was being fed by the one sitting on the opposite side. By helping one another, they helped themselves."

The point of this story is clear. It highlights Zig Ziglar's message: you can get everything in life you want, if you help enough people get what they want. If you want more love in your life, give more love. If you want more acceptance in your life, become more accepting of others. Whatever you want, you have to give it first before you can receive.

STEP 2. *Develop positive qualities*

What traits do you value in other people? What are the positive qualities of a friend? A very special friend of mine sent me a fax one day. He had come across a poem and wrote that it made him think of me. After reading the poem, I felt truly honored.

A Friend...
Someone with whom you can share your inner feelings...
knowing you won't be judged or rejected.
Someone who gives freely...
without expectation or motivation.
Someone who lets you be who you are...
if you want to change, it's up to you.
Someone who is there when you're hurting...
offering true tenderness.
Someone who sees your beauty...
your true beauty.
Someone who gives you space when it's needed...
without hesitation.

Someone who listens…
to what you are really saying.
Someone who will consider your different beliefs…
without judgment.
Someone whom you always feel close to…
even when they are far away.
Someone with whom you feel comfortable…
anytime, anywhere, doing anything.
A friend is a special gift…
to be cherished forever.

—*Datus*

We all need the love and acceptance of friends and family. In order to meet these needs, we must first develop the positive qualities of friendship within ourselves. In other words, in order to have a friend, we must first be a friend. Many of the qualities needed are stated in the poem above. Let me list some of the positive qualities I admire in people and strive to attain:

- Honesty
- Integrity
- Humility
- Dependability
- Loyalty
- Sincerity
- Enthusiasm
- Hard-working
- Open-mindedness
- A sense of humor
- Dedication

The great news is that these positive qualities can be learned or developed. Develop the characteristics of a true friend deep within you, and you will be blessed with very gratifying and rewarding relationships—ones that will nourish your body, mind, and soul.

STEP 3. *Learn to listen*

The quality of any relationship ultimately comes down to the quality of its communication. The biggest roadblock to effective communication in most relationships is poor listening skills. I really believe that "listening is loving." When we are truly listening, we are telling the person that he or she is important to us and that we respect and love him or her. Here are seven tips to good listening that I found easy to learn and quite useful.

TIP #1

Do not interrupt. Allow the person you are communicating with to really share his feelings and thoughts uninterrupted. Empathize with him, put yourself in his shoes. If you first seek to understand, you will find yourself being better understood.

Tip #2

Be an active listener. This means that you must act really interested in what the other person is communicating. Listen to what she is saying instead of thinking about your response. Ask questions to gain more information or clarify what she is telling you. Good questions open lines of communication.

Tip #3

Be a reflective listener. Restate or reflect back to the other person your interpretation of what he is telling you. This simple technique shows the other person that you are both listening and understanding what he is saying. Restating what you think is being said may cause some short-term conflict in some situations, but is certainly worth the risk. Just explain that you want to be certain you understand what he is trying to say.

Tip #4

Wait to speak until the person or people you want to communicate with are listening. If they are not ready to listen, no matter how well you communicate, your message will not be heard.

Tip #5

Don't try to talk over somebody. If you find yourself being interrupted, relax. Don't try to out-talk the other person. If you are courteous and allow him to speak, eventually (unless he is extremely rude), he will respond likewise. If he doesn't, point out to him that he is interrupting the communication process. You can only do this if you have been a good listener. Double standards in relationships seldom work.

Tip #6

Help the other person become an active listener. This can be done by asking her if she understood what you were communicating. Ask her to tell you what she heard. If she doesn't seem to be understanding what you are saying, keep after it until she does.

Don't be afraid of long silences. Human communication involves much more than words. Unfortunately, in many situations silence can make us feel uncomfortable, but a great deal can be communicated during silences. Relax. Some people need silence to collect their thoughts and feel safe in communicating. The important thing to remember during silence is that you must remain an active listener.

Step 4. *Find the good*

The way you see others has an effect on how you relate to them, how they view you, and how you view yourself. I urge you to become what Zig Ziglar calls a "good finder"—someone who looks for the good in other people or situations. In *See You at the Top*, Zig tells the story of an experiment conducted at Harvard University by Dr. Robert Rosenthal. A series of tests involving three groups of students and three groups of rats were conducted under the supervision of Dr. Rosenthal. He informed the first group of students, "You're in luck. You are going to be working with genius rats. These rats have been bred for intelligence and are extremely bright. They will run through the maze with great ease."

The second group was told, "Your rats are just average. They are not too bright, not too dumb, just a bunch of average rats. Don't expect too much from them, because they are just average."

The third group was told, "Your rats are really dumb. If they find the end of the maze, it will be purely by accident."

For the next six weeks, the students timed the performance of individual rats running through the maze. Not surprisingly, the genius rats behaved like geniuses and had the lowest times. The average rats were average and the dumb rats were really dumb.

What is so amazing about this study? Well, it turns out that all of the rats were from the same litter. There were no genius, average, or dumb rats. The only difference between them was the direct result of the difference in attitude and expectations of the students conducting the experiments.

Does the same thing happen with humans? Most definitely. Studies conducted with teachers and children produced the same kind of results as the studies with the rats. Remarkable as it may seem, it has been shown many times in controlled experiments that parents, teachers, managers, and others will get exactly what they expect. This phenomenon is called the "Pygmalion Effect."

According to Greek mythology, Pygmalion was a sculptor and King of Cyprus who fell in love with one of his creations. The ivory statue came to life after Pygmalion's repeated prayers to the Goddess of Love, Venus. Pygmalion's vision was so powerful and his faith so strong, his vision became his reality. The myth exemplifies the truth that what we see reflected in many objects, situations, or persons is what we put there with our own expectations. We create images of how things should be, and if these images are believed, they become self-fulfilling prophecies.

If we expect only the worst from people, that is exactly what we see. If we focus our attention on the positives, if we look for the good in people and situations, that becomes our reality. In addition, if we are constantly criticizing and looking for the negatives in people, this attitude is reflected. We too are harshly judged, criticized, and not very well liked.

To be happy and have positive relationships, you absolutely must become a good finder. You must look for the good in people. You must expect the best from people. And, you must reinforce the good that you see. You must demonstrate your love and appreciation.

STEP 5. *Demonstrate love and appreciation*

It is not enough to simply feel love in our friendships and intimate relationships. We must express these feelings. We must demonstrate to our loved ones just how important they are to us. We must continually find ways to communicate our deepest feelings through our actions, whether they be verbal, written, through touch, or by our behavior. We all need to see, hear, and physically feel loved and appreciated.

What are some ways to express love and appreciation? The most direct is to tell the person face-to-face or with a card or letter. Think of some times in your life when you felt really loved or appreciated. What made you feel that way? If a certain action produced a feeling of being loved and appreciated within you, it is likely that a similar action will produce those same feelings in another person. What a phenomenal gift you can give! I strongly urge you to seek out ways to continually tell those around you how much you love and appreciate them. Again, it is important to remember that what we give out, we get back.

STEP 6. *Develop intimacy*

Intimacy is very important to good health. It probably relates to the nurturing that takes place when we share our deepest selves. Intimate relationships are the most gratifying. However, many people have a hard time developing a truly intimate relationship—especially with their spouse. Friendships can be intimate, but our most intimate relationship is usually with our spouse or "significant other." The benefit here is that in addition to emotional intimacy, we also share physical intimacy.

Here are three simple tips to help nourish intimacy between friends or lovers:

Tip #1

Take a walk together. Moving together physically really opens up communication. It has to do with body language and a phenomenon called "mirroring and matching." Adopting another person's speech, body language, or behavior triggers our subconscious to develop a feeling of rapport. The next time you are out in a restaurant, take a look around and notice how many people (especially lovers) are mirroring and matching. You'll be amazed. Try using mirroring and matching to your advantage to enhance intimacy. It is very powerful.

Tip #2

Ask questions which open communication and let your partner answer the questions fully. This tip is extremely useful when challenges present themselves. The key is to frame questions in a positive light and allow your partner to really express him or herself. For example, when you ask your partner what kind of a day he or she had, listen to the feelings behind the words. Try to hear any concerns he or she might want to talk out. When something good happens, let your partner know how delighted you are for his success, how proud you are of her accomplishment. Let him or her expound. Really listen!

Tip #3

Find an activity that you both enjoy and do it together. Whether it is going to a movie, playing a game, eating at a favorite restaurant, or taking a drive or a walk together, it doesn't matter, as long as it is something you both enjoy doing, and you are doing it together.

If you have few intimate relationships in your life, you need to reach out and establish more friendships. Here are four additional tips you may find useful:

TIP #4

Look for opportunities to extend the contacts you make through your church, fitness center, or community program.

TIP #5

Attend workshops, seminars, and classes you are interested in. You will find people who share your beliefs and interests—fertile ground for developing supportive friendships.

TIP #6

Become a volunteer at your local hospital, school, nursing home, or any other place where you can really make a difference.

TIP #7

Get a pet. A relationship with a pet can be almost as positive as a human relationship. Studies have shown that owning or caring for a pet can relieve loneliness, depression, and anxiety, and even promote a quicker recovery from illness.

STEP 7. *Recognize challenges in relationships*

Any good relationship is going to be faced with challenges. It is from these challenges that the relationship will either be enhanced, nourished, and encouraged to grow—or be destroyed. A relationship based on love, trust, honesty, respect, and other positive values will survive any challenge; however, a relationship that lacks a strong foundation may crumble after even a very minor challenge.

Most challenges in relationships are the result of incomplete or misunderstood communications. In her book, *Making Love All of the Time,* Dr. Barbara De Angelis identifies four phases that can kill a relationship. By recognizing these four phases, you can prevent challenges from escalating to a level which can destroy the relationship. Here are the four phases:

Phase One—Resistance

The first phase of a relationship challenge is resistance. Resistance occurs when you take exception or feel annoyed or a bit separate from this person. It's nothing major, but if not effectively dealt with by loving communication, resistance can turn into resentment.

Phase Two—Resentment

The seed of resistance has flowered into a stronger negative feeling—resentment. You are not just annoyed; feelings of anger are present and an emotional barrier develops that destroys intimacy. If not dealt with, resentment then turns into rejection.

Phase Three—Rejection

In this phase, everything your partner does irritates or annoys you. Little meaningless things grow into huge conflicts. Rejection means emotional separation, yet it is quite painful. If not dealt with, rejection then turns into repression.

Phase Four—Repression

When you are tired of coping with the anger that comes with the rejection phase, repressing emotions becomes a mechanism to deal with the pain. Although pain is somewhat avoided, so is love, passion, and excitement. Couples become more like roommates than lovers in this phase.

Recognizing these four phases is the first step in preventing them from destroying a relationship. When you find yourself in one of these phases, it is critical to eliminate the negative feelings by addressing their source. Trying to sweep things under a rug or ignoring them only makes things worse.

The key to avoiding or getting out of this spiral of negative feelings is communication. Explain clearly the specific instance that is bothering you, but remember to ask questions in a positive light and really listen to your partner. Chances are both of you are feeling cut off, hurt, rejected. Try to empathize with the hurt inside your partner. When you listen with love and concern, doors open.

A relationship takes commitment from both parties. You must both be committed to learning how to communicate and behave in a manner consistent with your feelings. This small price is well worth the bounty of rewards that comes from positive relationships.

CHAPTER FOUR

KEY #4—A HEALTHY LIFESTYLE

STEP 1
Do not smoke

STEP 2
Drink only in moderation or do not drink at all

STEP 3
Get adequate rest

STEP 4
Learn to deal with stress effectively

STEP 5
Learn to manage time effectively

STEP 6
Connect with nature

STEP 7
Laugh long and often

Key #4—A Healthy Lifestyle

It is no secret that lifestyle choices—particularly smoking, excessive use of alcohol, and diet/nutrition—are preventable risk factors for many of the leading causes of death in the United States. In fact, Americans younger than age 65 have higher chances of dying from preventable conditions than residents of other industrialized nations. The United States has also made the least improvement in reducing preventable deaths, when compared to other countries.

Babies born in 2009 (the most recent data available) have a life expectancy of 76 years for boys, and 80.9 years for girls. However, by making better choices earlier in life, life expectancy can increase, and perhaps more importantly, the number of healthy years in your life can increase.

Step 1. *Do not smoke*

Cigarette smoking is one of the major factors contributing to premature death in the United States. Health experts have determined that cigarette smoking is the single major cause of cancer death in the United States. Cigarette smokers have total, overall cancer death rates twice that of non-smokers. The greater the number of cigarettes smoked, the greater the risk.

Smoking also increases the risk of death from heart attacks and strokes. In fact, according to the U.S. Surgeon General, "Cigarette smoking should be considered the most important risk factor for coronary heart disease." Statistical evidence reveals a three-to-fivefold increase in the risk of coronary artery disease in smokers compared to non-smokers. The more cigarettes smoked and the longer a person has smoked, the greater the risk of dying from a heart attack or stroke. Overall, the average smoker dies seven to eight years sooner than the non-smoker.

If you want good health, you absolutely must stop smoking! Here are eleven tips to help you stop:

Tip #1
List all the reasons why you want to quit smoking and
review them daily.

Tip #2
Set a specific day to quit, tell at least ten friends that you are
going to quit smoking, and then DO IT!

Tip #3

Throw away all cigarettes, butts, matches, and ashtrays.

Tip #4

Use substitutes. Instead of smoking, chew on raw vegetables, fruits, or gum. If your fingers seem empty, play with a pencil.

Tip #5

Take one day at a time.

Tip #6

Realize that more than 40 million Americans have quit. If they can do it, so can you!

Tip #7

Visualize yourself as a non-smoker with a fatter pocketbook, pleasant breath, unstained teeth, and the satisfaction that comes from being in control of your life.

Tip #8

Join a support group. Call the local American Cancer Society and ask for referrals. You are not alone.

Tip #9

When you need to relax, perform deep breathing exercises rather than reaching for a cigarette.

Tip #10

Avoid situations that you associate with smoking.

Tip #11

Each day, reward yourself in a positive way. Buy yourself something with the money you've saved or plan a special reward as a celebration for quitting

STEP 2. *Drink only in moderation or do not drink*

Alcohol is our nation's number one drug problem. In fact, according to the National Institutes of Health, 18 million Americans (7% of the population) are dependent on alcohol or have problems related to the use of alcohol.

While moderate drinking (no more than one or two drinks per day) has actually been shown to be associated with a longer life, excessive drinking is strongly associated with five of the leading causes of death in the United States: accidents, cirrhosis of the liver, pneumonia, suicide, and murder.

Consequences of alcohol abuse
Increased mortality:
- 10-year decrease in life expectancy
- Double the usual death rate in men, triple in women
- Six times greater suicide rate
- Major contributing factor in the four leading causes of death in men between the ages of 25 and 44: accidents, homicides, suicides, cirrhosis

Economic toll (yearly):
- Lost production: over $20 billion
- Health care costs: over $10 billion
- Accident and fire losses: $5 billion
- Cost of violent crime: $4 billion

Health effects:
- Metabolic damage to every cell
- Intoxication
- Abstinence and withdrawal syndromes
- Nutritional diseases
- Brain damage
- Psychiatric disorders
- Esophagitis, gastritis, ulcer
- Increased cancer of mouth, pharynx, larynx, esophagus
- Pancreatitis
- Liver fatty degeneration and cirrhosis
- Heart disease
- High blood pressure
- Angina
- Hypoglycemia
- Decreased protein synthesis
- Increased serum and liver triglycerides
- Decreased serum testosterone
- Muscle damage
- Osteoporosis
- Birth defects

If you think you have a drinking problem, seek out help. Contact your local Alcoholics Anonymous or similar program. Also, I have found that many people with alcoholism have faulty control over blood sugar levels. People who crave sugar and alcohol can benefit by eating small, frequent meals and taking a nutritional formula that provides essential nutrients required by the body to regulate blood sugar levels.

STEP 3. *Get adequate rest*

Are you getting enough sleep? If not, your health may be suffering. Sufficient sleep and rest are essential to good health. Your body needs sleep to function properly. During sleep, the body repairs itself. Without sufficient sleep, needed repairs go undone, and the body is more likely to break down.

During sleep, your body systems undergo major positive changes. For example:

- Brain waves slow down
- Blood pressure falls
- Muscles relax
- The pituitary gland produces more hormones
- Immune function is enhanced
- Your body actively repairs damaged tissues and cells
- You dream, allowing your mind to work out unresolved psychological and emotional issues

Exactly how much sleep you need depends upon you. Some people find they need only 5 or 6 hours of sleep; others may need 10 or 11. Regardless of how much sleep you think you might require, the truth is most Americans do not get enough sleep to function optimally. In addition, at least 40 million Americans suffer from insomnia or some other sleep disturbance.

To improve your ability to sleep, give yourself some time to wind down before going to bed. Avoid stimulants such as caffeine or television programs that keep you on the edge of your seat. Sip some herbal tea and listen to some beautiful music or a relaxation tape. Let the day go. Whatever you must accomplish tomorrow, give yourself permission to rest now, so you'll wake with the energy needed to get the job done.

STEP 4. *Learn to deal with stress effectively*

Stress is common in our fast-paced society. Often, the demands placed on us daily build until it is almost impossible to cope. Job pressures. Family arguments. Financial pressures. Deadlines. These are common examples of "stressors." Actually, a stressor can be anything that creates a disturbance within our body: exposure to heat or cold, environmental toxins, toxins produced by micro-organisms, physical trauma, and, of course, strong emotions.

Some basic control mechanisms are geared toward counteracting the everyday stresses of life. The initial response to stress is the alarm reaction, or "flight or fight" response. Triggered by reactions in the brain which cause the adrenal glands to secrete adrenaline and other stress-related hormones, the fight or flight response is designed to counteract danger by mobilizing the body's resources for immediate physical activity. This is great if you need to escape from a tiger or some other life-threatening situation. However, if stress is extreme, unusual, or long-lasting, the effects of these mechanisms can be quite harmful.

Conditions strongly linked to psychological stress
- Angina
- Asthma
- Autoimmune disease
- Cancer
- Cardiovascular disease
- Common cold
- Depression
- Diabetes (adult onset, Type II)
- Headaches
- Hypertension
- Immune system suppression
- Irritable bowel
- Menstrual syndrome irregularities
- Premenstrual tension
- Rheumatoid arthritis syndrome
- Ulcerative colitis
- Ulcers

Specific relaxation techniques can reduce the amount of stress. (For example, I have described a relaxation/visualization exercise on pages 29 and 30.) Even more important than the *type* of relaxation technique is that you set aside at least 10 to 15 minutes each day to do it.

Although you can relax by simply sleeping, watching television, or reading a book, certain relaxation techniques are designed specifically to produce the physiological state Herbert Benson, M.D., describes in his best-selling book, *The Relaxation Response*. The physiological effects of the relaxation response are opposite those seen with stress.

In the stress response, the sympathetic nervous system dominates. In the relaxation response, the parasympathetic nervous system dominates. The parasympathetic nervous system controls body functions such as digestion, breathing, and heart rate during periods of rest, relaxation, visualization, meditation, and sleep. While the sympathetic nervous system is designed to protect us against immediate danger, the parasympathetic system is designed for repair, maintenance, and restoration of the body.

Producing deep relaxation with any relaxation technique requires learning how to breathe. Have you ever noticed how a baby breathes? With each breath, the baby's abdomen rises and falls because the baby is breathing with its diaphragm, a dome-shaped muscle that separates the chest cavity from the abdominal cavity. If you are like most adults, you tend to fill only your upper chest because you do not utilize the diaphragm. Shallow breathing tends to produce tension and fatigue.

One of the most powerful methods of producing less stress and more energy in the body is breathing with the diaphragm. By using the diaphragm to breathe, you can dramatically change your physiology. Diaphragmatic breathing literally activates the relaxation centers in the brain. Here is a popular technique I use to train people to breathe using their diaphragm.

- Find a quiet, comfortable place to lie down or sit.
- Place your feet slightly apart. Place one hand on your abdomen near your navel. Place the other hand on your chest.
- You will be inhaling through your nose and exhaling through your mouth.
- Concentrate on your breathing. Note which hand is rising and falling with each breath.
- Gently exhale most of the air in your lungs.
- Inhale while slowly counting to 4. As you inhale, slightly extend your abdomen, causing it to rise about one inch. Make sure that you are not moving your chest or shoulders.
- As you inhale, imagine the warmed air flowing in. Imagine its warmth flowing to all parts of your body.
- Pause for one second, then slowly exhale to a count of 4. As you exhale, your abdomen should move inward.
- As the air flows out, imagine all the tension and stress leaving your body.
- Repeat the process until a sense of deep relaxation is achieved.

Now that you know how to breathe, the important thing is to remember to breathe with your diaphragm as much as possible—especially during times of increased stress—and perform a relaxation technique for 10 to 15 minutes each day.

STEP 5. *Learn to manage time effectively*

One of the biggest stressors for most people is time—they simply do not feel they have enough of it. Here are some tips on time management that really seem to work. Oh, by the way, time management does not mean squeezing more and more work into less and less time. It means learning to plan your time more effectively, so you can do the activities in life that you enjoy.

TIP #1

Set priorities. Realize that you can only accomplish so much in a day. Decide what is important, and limit your efforts to that goal.

TIP #2

Organize your day. Interruptions and unplanned demands on your time will always occur, but create a definite plan for the day based on your priorities. Avoid the pitfall of allowing the "immediate demands" to control your life.

TIP #3

Delegate authority. Delegate as much authority and work as you can. You can't do everything yourself. Learn to train and depend on others.

TIP #4

Tackle the toughest job first. Handle the most important tasks first while your energy levels are high. Leave the busywork or running around for later in the day.

TIP #5

Minimize meeting time. Schedule meetings to bump up against the lunch hour or quitting time; that way they can't last forever.

Tip #6

Avoid putting things off. Work done under pressure of an unreasonable deadline often has to be redone. That creates more stress than if it had been done right the first time. Plan ahead.

Tip #7

Don't be a perfectionist. You can never really achieve perfection anyway. Do your best in a reasonable amount of time, then move on to other important tasks. If you find time, you can always come back later and polish the task some more.

Step 6. *Connect with nature*

Most Americans spend 90% of their lives indoors separated from fresh air, natural sunlight, and nature. Something extremely refreshing and calming happens when we can get in touch with nature, whether it is simply a walk through a park or getting out in the wilderness for a weekend of camping. Personally, I find the rhythms and sounds of nature very relaxing. Since I can't always get out and enjoy nature as much as I would like, I do the next best thing—I listen to sounds of nature.

In my office, car, and home, I usually have a recording of sounds of nature playing in the background. The recordings are of beautifully relaxing music intertwined with sounds of nature, like the sounds at an isolated beach, waterfall, or forest. I find myself being more productive and relaxed when these gentle sounds are playing. I highly recommend it.

Step 7. *Laugh long and often*

The late Norman Cousins' popular book *Anatomy of an Illness* caused a significant stir in the medical community in 1979. Cousins' book provided an autobiographical anecdotal account of how laughter and positive emotional states can help heal the body, even of quite serious disease. Cousins watched Candid Camera and Marx Brothers films, and read humorous books.

Originally, physicians and researchers scoffed at Cousins' account. Now, however, numerous studies have demonstrated that laughter and other positive emotional states can, in fact, enhance the immune system. Recent medical research has also confirmed that laughter:

- enhances blood flow to the body's extremities and improves cardiovascular function,
- plays an active part in the body's release of endorphins and other natural mood-elevating and pain-killing chemicals, and
- improves the transfer of oxygen and nutrients to internal organs.

By laughing frequently and taking a lighter view of life, you will find that life is much more enjoyable and fun. Here are eight tips to help you get more laughter in your life.

Tip #1

Learn to laugh at yourself.

Recognize how funny some of your behavior really is—especially your shortcomings or mistakes. I am really lucky because I have many little foibles and goofs that make me laugh at myself. And, I work at EuroPharma®, a great place where people accept me for who I am, but can point out little things I do that are funny.

For example, I have trouble saying certain words. When I say specific, it comes out "pecific." I don't know why or how it comes out this way, but it almost always does. Most people wouldn't even notice, but at staff meetings when I am talking about a product which is derived from a "pecific" fraction of bovine liver—it seems everyone notices and gets a good laugh in, including myself. Hey, we are all human. We all have little idiosyncrasies or behaviors that are unique to us that we can recognize and enjoy.

I must point out that there is a big difference between laughing with others and laughing at others. Because of the atmosphere at EuroPharma and the values of the company and its employees, I know that when I say "pecific," people are not laughing at me, they are laughing with me. I am included in the laughter because I can laugh at myself. In fact, now that I am aware of it, I will often exaggerate and say that our product is from a "pecific" fraction of bovine liver just to lighten up the mood of a meeting.

Tip #2

Inject humor anytime it is appropriate.

I just gave an example of injecting humor into a meeting. At EuroPharma, humor abounds. Consultants who come into our offices are amazed at how productive our staff is and how much they seem to be enjoying their work. They are amazed to sit in on our executive meetings and observe us laughing regularly, yet still accomplishing our meeting goals. I explain to them that I believe we are accomplishing our goals and objectives so well because of our enjoyment of each other and the whole process.

Humor and laughter really make work enjoyable. We have employees who cannot wait to get to work because they have so much fun in their jobs. I want my employees to be happy. I believe they have to be free to inject humor into their work in order to be happy. They have the freedom to socialize and share among themselves as long as they get their work done. While some managers might look at such behavior as "goofing off," I recognize the importance of humor in developing good morale and greater productivity.

Tip #3

Find a humor-based website and read it often.

A joke a day can help put a smile on your face. There are quit a few websites that run syndicated cartoons or publish a humerous joke or story of the day. Find a site you like and check it often for a pick-me-up when you need a chuckle.

Tip #4

Watch comedies on television.

With modern cable systems, I am amazed at how easy it is to find something funny on television. When I am in need of a good laugh, I try to find something I can laugh at on TV. Some of my favorites are the old-time classics like Andy Griffith, Gilligan's Island, Mary Tyler Moore, etc. If I can't find anything on TV, or the comedies are too mean spirited, then I will watch something from my DVD collection. I have collected all of the Andy Griffith shows because no matter how many times I see an episode, it always makes me laugh or feel good inside.

Tip #5

Go to comedies at the movie theater.

I love to go to the movies, especially a comedy. It is not just my personal enjoyment of the movie that I like. What I enjoy most is going to the movie with my family or friends because their companionship really enhances the whole experience. If we see a funny movie together, I find myself laughing harder and longer. We feed off each other's laughter during and after the movie. Sharing a funny movie together means that we will be talking about specific (there is that word again) scenes from the movie that really made us laugh.

Tip #6

Listen to comedy DVDs or a humorous radio show in your car.

Check your local record or book store, video store, or library for recorded comedy routines of your favorite comic. If you haven't heard or seen many comics, go to your library first. You'll find an abundance of CDs to investigate, and you can check them out for free.

Tip #7

Play with kids.

Kids really know how to laugh and play. If you do not have kids of your own, spend time with your nieces, nephews, or neighborhood children with whose families you are friendly. Become a Big Brother or Big Sister. Investigate local Little Leagues. Help out at your church's Sunday School and children's events.

Tip #8

Ask yourself, "What is funny about this situation?"

Many times we will find ourselves in seemingly impossible situations, but, if we can laugh about them, somehow they become enjoyable or at least tolerable experiences. One time, I was visiting some companies in Europe with a colleague, and we found ourselves in an interesting situation. We had gotten on an express train going in the opposite direction of where we were supposed to be headed. Express trains are so- called because they only make stops at large cities many miles apart.

Our immediate reaction was to break out into almost uncontrollable laughter. We immediately recognized the humor of our situation and realized we were powerless to stop the train and turn it around. We could only accept our mistake, wait for the next stop (about an hour), and board a new train going in the right direction.

Some people would have become angry or started asking negative questions like, "How could we be so stupid?" or "What did we do to deserve this?" Or, they would have tried to delegate blame. Instead of a "negative" experience, we were given another experience that we can reflect back on with a good laugh.

So many times, I have heard people say, "This is something you will look back on and laugh about." Well, why wait—find the humor in the situation and enjoy a good laugh immediately.

Chapter Five

Key #5—Regular Exercise

Step 1
Realize the importance of physical exercise

Step 2
Consult your physician

Step 3
Choose an exercise program

Step 4
Short burst exercise

Step 5
Do it often

Step 6
Make it fun

Step 7
Stay motivated

Key #5—Regular Exercise

Regular exercise is vital to good health. We all know this fact, yet only about half of Americans report they exercise regularly (at least three sessions a week). Why? Excuses like lack of time, energy, or motivation are frequently given. How valid are these excuses? How important is your health? How important is regular exercise to your overall health?

Exercise is absolutely essential to achieving optimal health. While the immediate effect of exercise is perceived as a stress on the body, with regular exercise the body adapts—it becomes stronger, functions more efficiently, and has greater endurance. Your entire body benefits from regular exercise, largely as a result of improved cardiovascular and respiratory functions. Simply stated, exercise boosts the transport of oxygen and nutrients into cells. At the same time, exercise enhances the transport of carbon dioxide and waste products from the tissues of the body to the bloodstream and ultimately to the eliminative organs. As a result, regular exercise increases stamina and energy levels.

Physical inactivity is a major reason so many Americans are over-weight. This is especially true in children. Studies have demonstrated that childhood obesity is associated more with inactivity than overeating. Since strong evidence suggests that 80-86% of adult obesity begins in childhood, it can be concluded that lack of physical activity is a major cause of obesity.

Regular exercise is a necessary component of any effective weight-loss program due to the following factors:

1. When weight loss is achieved *without* exercise, a substantial portion of total weight loss comes from lean tissue, primarily as water loss. However, when exercise *is* included in a weight-loss program, body composition improves. Lean body weight increases because of an increase in muscle mass and a decrease in body fat. Since muscle burns calories, an increase in muscle mass means your body is burning more calories all day long – even while you're asleep.
2. Exercise helps counter the reduction in your basal metabolic rate (the rate at which your body burns calories at rest) that occurs as we age. In fact, exercise can increase basal metabolic rate not only when you're exercising, but for an extended period of time following the exercise session.
3. Moderate to intense exercise may help to suppress the appetite.

People who exercise during and after weight reduction are better able to maintain their weight loss than those who do not exercise.

Regular exercise also exerts a powerful positive effect on the mind. Tension, depression, feelings of inadequacy, and worries tend to diminish with regular exercise. Research has demonstrated that exercise can have a tremendous impact on improving mood and the ability to handle life's stressful situations.

In fact, a study published in the *American Journal of Epidemiology* found that increased participation in exercise, sports, and physical activities is strongly associated with decreased symptoms of anxiety (restlessness, tension, etc.), depression (feeling that life is not worthwhile, low spirits, etc.), and malaise (rundown feeling, insomnia, etc.). Simply stated, people who participate in regular exercise have higher self-esteem, feel better, and are happier.

This is due to the ability of regular exercise to enhance powerful mood-elevating substances in the brain known as endorphins. These compounds exert effects similar to morphine. In fact, their name (endo = endogenous, -rphins = morphine) was given to them because of their morphine-like effects. A clear association exists between exercise and endorphin elevation—when endorphins go up, mood follows.

Dennis Lobstein, Ph.D., a professor of exercise physiology at the University of New Mexico, compared the beta-endorphin levels and depression profiles of 10 joggers versus 10 sedentary men of the same age. The ten sedentary men tested as more depressed, perceived greater stress in their lives, had more stress-circulating hormones, and showed lower levels of beta-endorphins. As Dr. Lobstein stated, this "reaffirms that depression is very sensitive to exercise and helps firm up a biochemical link between physical activity and depression."

If the benefits of exercise could be put in a pill, you would have the most powerful health-promoting medication available. Take a look at this long list of health benefits produced by regular exercise:

Musculoskeletal System
- Increases muscle strength
- Increases lean body mass
- Increases muscle flexibility and range of motion
- Produces strong bones, ligaments, and tendons
- Helps improve calcium deposition in bones
- Prevents osteoporosis

- Lessens chance of injury
- Enhances posture, poise, and physique

Cardiovascular System
- Lowers resting heart rate
- Strengthens heart function
- Lowers blood pressure
- Improves oxygen delivery throughout the body
- Increases blood supply to muscles
- Enlarges the arteries to the heart
- Reduces heart disease risk
- Raises HDL, the "good" cholesterol
- Helps balance blood cholesterol and triglycerides

Bodily Processes
- Improves immune function
- Aids digestion and elimination
- Improves the body's ability to burn dietary fat
- Increases endurance and energy levels
- Improves sensitivity to insulin
- Reduces risk of diabetes

Mental Processes
- Provides a natural release for pent-up feelings
- Helps reduce tension and anxiety
- Improves mental outlook and self-esteem
- Helps relieve moderate depression
- Improves the ability to handle stress
- Stimulates improved mental function
- Relaxes and improves sleep

Longevity
Research shows that for every hour we exercise, we gain a two-hour increase in longevity.

STEP 1. *Realize the importance of physical exercise*
My own path to exercise started in my teens and early 20's. At 5'7" tall, my weight had ballooned to 250 pounds. I enlisted in the Marine Corps, where I was encouraged—ok, maybe *forced* is a better word—to work out.

My daily exercise regimen consisted of obstacle courses and 10-mile runs. During the same time a captain in the Marine Corps mentored me in weight lifting and physical exercise and introduced me to my first health food store in Oceanside, California. The lifestyle that I adopted then eventually brought me to where I am today—healthy, at an appropriate weight, and with a better understanding about health and nutrition. It changed **my** whole life. Now I hope I can help you change **your** life.

Step 2. *Consult your physician*

If you are not currently participating in a regular exercise program, I recommend consulting with your healthcare practitioner (especially if you have health problems or are over 40 years of age) prior to starting an exercise program. The main concern is your heart function. Exercise can be quite harmful (even fatal) if your heart is not able to meet the increased demands placed upon it. It is especially important to see a physician if any of the following applies to you:

- Heart disease
- Smoking
- High blood pressure
- Extreme breathlessness with physical exertion
- Pain or pressure in the chest, arms (especially left arm), teeth, jaw, or neck with exercise
- Dizziness or fainting
- Abnormal heart action (palpitations or irregular heartbeat)

Step 3. *Choose an exercise program*

If you are fit enough to begin, the next thing to do is select an activity that you feel you would enjoy. People are always asking which activity is the best kind of exercise. **The best kind is the one that gets you moving and your heart pumping.** Traditional forms of aerobic exercise, such as walking briskly, jogging, bicycling, cross-country skiing, swimming, aerobic dance, and racquet sports are good examples.

Through the years I tried to maintain a traditional exercise program that consisted of running for cardiovascular conditioning, along with additional weight lifting. I was doing about 1-1 ½ hours three to four times a week. While I received good benefit from this traditional form of exercise, it was just too time consuming.

I found that I just could not afford the time I was devoting to working out. I'm sure many of you can identify—often times, daily life leaves little to no time for exercise. I decided then and there to search for a form of exercise that could give me a full body workout, including cardiovascular, in a limited amount of time.

In my search, I ran across information on kettle bell training. I kept seeing mention of an exercise program designed by Dr. Al Sears called PACE. I was also made aware of it by a good friend, Dr. Jonathan Wright. If you've never seen a kettle bell, it looks like a cannonball with a handle and weighs anywhere from 5 to 106 lbs.

My goal was to give me and my 400+ muscles, including the most important muscle, my heart, a vigorous workout in the shortest period of time. I started working out on my own with the kettle bells, doing a 12-20 minute routine two or three times a week. Over the course of two years I was able to stay in very good shape and did not lose the benefits of my prior exercise routine where I was spending 1-1½ hours on each work out. It was proof that I could stay as fit as before but on *1/3 or less* the time that I had been devoting to exercise. This is a routine that everybody can do. You select the type of exercise and the degree of intensity. Combine that with a rest period in between the exercises and you have the entire program.

STEP 4. *Short burst exercise—An efficient and effective option*

When it comes to exercise, I think we really need to take a cue from the animal kingdom. Most animals who are strong and powerful do not run long distances, but rather maintain their power and strength by using short bursts of energy to either capture their next meal or escape from being some other animal's next meal.

I'm not an advocate for long distance running (marathons). Although this may be a sport, it's not a healthy one, and in fact it is actually very damaging to the muscles, particularly the heart. Take a look at runners who sprint with short bursts and then rest. They tend to have lean, muscular, healthy-looking bodies. People who run marathons will lose weight but tend to also lose muscle tone, and are found to have a higher body fat to lean muscle ratio. An old acquaintance, a young man in his late 20's—very active running marathons and playing tennis—was about 5'8" and weighed around 145 pounds but had a body fat ratio to lean muscle of 24%. Although slim and lean, he was a good candidate for a heart attack.

Running a marathon creates an inflammatory storm in the body that is identical to the early symptoms of heart disease. In his research, Dr. Sears notes one study in particular which found that 35% of marathoners had significant levels of arterial plaque compared to just 22% of non-marathon runners. That's an increased risk of over 50%. Dr. Sears also points to the Harvard Health Professionals Study which found the key to lowering heart disease risk is the intensity of the exercise—not repetition, endurance and duration.

As mentioned earlier, long distance running is very damaging because it creates large quantities of free radicals and inflammation. Heart attacks are just as common in long distance runners as they are in sedentary people. If you are an individual who enjoys running and wants to continue running marathons, I would encourage you to use a strong antioxidant supplement like curcumin (see Chapter 7, Step 2), which has very powerful anti-inflammatory, pain-relieving and antioxidant properties.

Developed in the 1960's by Dr. Per Asrand, the term fatrtlek, meaning "speed play", described the type of short burst training (SBT) used by the Swedes. The major benefits of interval training, or "SBT", include raising levels of human growth hormone, burning more calories, tapping into the strength of large muscle fibers, and developing more muscle and strength and greater fitness in less time.

Additional scientific studies have provided further documentation that a short workout routine with emphasis on high intensity and ample rest in between could accomplish more than a long, slow paced form of exercise.

A study at Laval University in Quebec divided participants into two groups: a long duration exercise group and an interval short term exercise group. They had the long duration group cycle up to 45 minutes without interruption. The short term interval group cycled in numerous short bursts of 15-90 seconds while resting in between. The long duration group burned twice as many calories so you would assume they would burn more fat. However, when the researchers recorded their body composition measurements, the interval group showed they lost the most fat. **In fact, the interval group lost *nine times* more fat than the endurance group for every calorie burned.**

Researchers following over 7,000 people in the large Harvard Health Professionals Study found that the key to exercise is not length or endurance. **It's intensity.** The more energy a person exerted, the lower their risk of heart disease. High intensity exercise can also help you live longer. Another Harvard Study compared vigorous and light exercise. Those who performed more vigorous exercise had a lower risk of death than those who performed less vigorous exercise.

I have researched and personally benefitted from intense, short burst exercise. My 12-20 minute exercise program consists of using a series of kettle bell swings and a stationary recumbent bike. I use either a 44 lb or 53 lb kettle bell and do a kettle bell swing 30-35 times, which takes about 20-30 seconds and is like running 200 meters as fast as you can. I then do a two minute "rest" following the intense burst of activity. My two minutes of rest refers to pedaling (usually at the lowest level) on a recumbent bike. I call this active rest and it is done in order to provide continued circulation of the blood and facilitate removal of lactic acid from the muscles. Depending on the level of fitness, people can start off with a 5 lb kettle bell or whatever is most suitable. Women will find the 5 or 10 lb kettle bell more than enough. Men may want to do 10 or 20 lbs for a good exercise regimen.

You want to continue doing the swing until you can no longer breathe and then take a two minute rest. Repeat this sequence five or six times or as long as it takes to do in a period of 12-20 minutes. Some people do the kettle bell swing for 30-35 swings, and then for their rest period they jump rope for two minutes. I can't for the life of me jump rope, so I use the recumbent bike as an active rest period. It is never a good idea to sit down for your rest period. You want to continue moving or walking around or bouncing on your feet. No matter what your day is like, I think everyone can find 12-20 minutes three or four times a week.

Even if you can only begin exercising and doing a kettle bell swing using a 10 ounce can of peas, that would be a good place to start. As you progress, you can slowly increase your intensity. Case in point: In one of Dr. Sears' most severe cases, he worked with a lady who started off walking for 45 seconds and then rested two minutes and walked an additional 45 seconds and continued this process. Altogether she lost over 60 pounds and was in much better health and had nice muscle tone. The whole idea is to exercise for 20-30 seconds at your highest level of intensity.

Remember, you are only competing against yourself—so work as hard as you can at some form of exercise for 20-30 seconds. For me it's the kettle bells. For others it may be sprinting or swimming 100 yards as fast as you can with a two minute rest. This is repeated until you have your 12-20 minutes in. I believe everyone can do this. I challenge you to use my menu plan and this exercise program for a minimum of six months and watch the unbelievable results you'll achieve. I will give you a few websites that I think you should explore so you can learn more:

- www.alsearsmd.com
- www.dragondoor.com
- www.artofstrength.com
- www.kettleworx.com

STEP 5. *Do it often*

You don't get in good physical condition by exercising just once. Exercise must be performed on a regular basis. A minimum of 12 to 20 minutes of exercise, 3-4 times a week is necessary to gain any significant cardiovascular benefits.

STEP 6. *Make it fun*

The key to getting the maximum benefit from exercise is to make it enjoyable. Choose an activity that you enjoy—whether it be swimming, racquetball, or kettle bells—and have fun! If you can find enjoyment in exercise, you are much more likely to do it regularly. One way to make it fun is to get a workout partner. Having an exercise buddy also keeps you accountable. The next time you contemplate backing out of a scheduled workout, you will realize you are not just letting yourself down, but your buddy as well.

STEP 7. *Stay motivated*

No matter how committed a person is to regular exercise, at some point, he or she will lose enthusiasm for working out. Here is my suggestion— take a break. Not a long break, just skip one or two workouts. Give your enthusiasm and motivation a chance to recoup, so you can come back with an even stronger commitment.

Here are some things I do to keep myself motivated:
- Read or thumb through fitness magazines like *Men's Fitness* and *Muscle & Fitness.* Looking at pictures of people in fantastic shape really inspires me. In addition, these magazines typically feature articles on interesting new exercise tips/routines I can incorporate into my own personal exercise routine.
- Set exercise goals. Since I am a goal-oriented individual, goals really help keep me motivated. Success breeds success, so make a lot of small goals that can easily be achieved. Write down your daily exercise goal and check it off when you have completed it.
- Vary your routine. Variety is important to keep exercise interesting. Doing the same thing every day becomes monotonous and drains motivation. Continually find new ways to enjoy working out.

Keep a record of your activities and progress. Sometimes it is hard to see the progress you are making but, if you write in a journal, you'll have a permanent record of your progress. Seeing your progress in black and white will motivate you to continued improvement.

CHAPTER SIX

KEY #6—A HEALTH-PROMOTING DIET

STEP 1
Ignore the "experts"

STEP 2
Get good quality protein every day

STEP 3
Include healthy fats in your diet

STEP 4
Boost intake of fruits and vegetables

STEP 5
Eat local and organic whenever possible

STEP 6
Avoid carbohydrates, sugar, and processed foods

STEP 7
Take time for meal planning

Key #6—A Health-Promoting Diet

Step 1. *Ignore the "experts"*

Want to live a long, healthy life? Ignore the "experts"!

I'm serious. The people who have told you to stop eating red meat, butter, and other nutritionally vital whole foods are just flat out wrong. If you look back to the kinds of diets that most Americans had in the 1940s or 1950s, according to popular belief *everyone* should have been overweight. Of course, that's not true. Older photographs or old movies shows how much thinner people were in the past compared to where we are now—with our carbohydrate-heavy diets, mistakenly recommended by medical experts in an effort to avoid fats.

The result isn't just people being overweight, but being sick and exhausted all of the time, having high blood pressure and the explosion of Type 2 diabetes. It's no wonder. Without animal proteins and fats, the body just doesn't get the nutrients it needs to survive and thrive. Whole foods and whole fats are what we are supposed to be eating! No wonder people feel hungry when they try to get by on processed "lite" diets—there's no nutrition there!

The picture this paints for the future isn't a good one. By 2030, obesity rates will increase another 8%, to include 42% of Americans, so almost half of Americans will be at least 30 lbs. overweight. The percentage of those who are severely obese (more than 100 lbs. overweight) is expected to be 11% by 2030—double the current rate. Unfortunately, we learn habits—good and bad—early. In cases of obesity, that's sadly the case. In fact, 50% of those who are severely obese as adults were also obese as children.

For centuries, the original and traditional diet for everyone—and the way some people still choose to eat today, including myself—was approximately 30% animal protein, 60% animal fat and 10% non-starchy carbohydrates. And that 10% of carbohydrates should be from fruits and vegetables. This is the diet I recommend for everyone. If you eat following these guidelines, consuming the foods I recommend below, I guarantee you will be thinner and healthier than ever before!

Step 2. *Get good proteins every day*

Protein is our original "power food" and it is absolutely necessary. I'd like to share my favorite food sources for great protein, and why they should definitely be a part of your diet. Remember that animal protein (which should make up approximately 30% of your diet) is rich in readily-absorbable amino acids, which are the building blocks of our brains and bodies. I highly encourage you to consider protein such as beef, poultry, bison, fish, seafood and eggs in place of the carbohydrate-rich diet you are probably currently consuming. Personally, I eat grass-fed beef, organic whenever possible, as it is naturally rich in omega-3 fatty acids. Remember—there were no feed lots in the Paleolithic age! While you should avoid smoked and processed meats, beef bacon is a healthier choice. Produced without cancer-causing nitrites, natural beef bacon can be rich in omega-3s (from grass-fed beef) and conjugated linoleic acids (CLAs). It makes a great substitute for overly processed pork bacon. Look for it at your health food store.

Seafood such as shrimp is rich in vitamin D, selenium, tryptophan, and B-12. Cold water fish like salmon are rich in omega-3 fatty acids, B12, niacin, vitamin D, and tryptophan, to name just a few nutrients. Salmon is also an excellent source of protein. If you're not a regular eater of seafood, (and I have to admit that I'm not) I urge you to get your omega-3s through supplementation (see Chapter 7 for specifics).

One of the big disasters of the "battle against cholesterol" has been disinformation about eggs. They are one of the best—and most reasonable —sources of protein and healthy fats available, and it is a shame nutrition "experts" have warned people away from them for so long. Eggs should be a part of your protein-rich diet. They provide vitamin B2, tryptophan, selenium, and are another source of iodine.

I think eggs from free-range producers are some of the best. If you or your family raised chickens for their eggs when you were young, you probably remember how great they tasted. The diet and living conditions of the hens really make a difference that your taste buds—and your health—will recognize.

Nuts are an excellent source of protein and healthy fats. And two that should absolutely be a part of your diet are almonds and walnuts. Almonds are a must for anyone who wants to lose weight and reduce their risk of heart disease. They are loaded with folate, plant sterols, fiber, vitamin E and magnesium. And while almonds do contain fat, 78% of the calories come from healthy, monounsaturated fats that help build strong cells and keep arteries flexible.

If you are dealing with a few extra pounds, consider almonds as the perfect snack. One study found that overweight people on a low-calorie diet plus 2.5 ounces of almonds daily lost 62% more weight, 50% more belly fat, and reduced their blood pressure by 11 points versus the control group eating low-calorie food and foods equal to the almonds for calories and protein.

Walnuts are an amazing source of many nutrients, including vitamin E (in gamma-tocopherol form), phenolic acids, alpha-linoleic acid, copper, manganese, and of course, protein. Walnuts are incredibly heart-friendly. Studies show that they improve vasodilation (relaxing of blood vessels and arteries) for individuals with diabetes, who are at greater risk of heart disease.

There are lots of healthy options out there to increase your protein intake. You will be amazed at how good, and good for you, they are!

STEP 3. *Include healthy fats in your diet*

The fear of fat has led to an epidemic of diseases that have occurred primarily because we have *reversed* the ratio of our food groups from high animal protein/animal fat and low carbohydrates, to high carbs and little or no healthy animal protein and animal fats. In fact, many Americans are consuming 60% to 70% of their meals as carbohydrates (mostly refined and processed), and 20% to 30% *unhealthy* fats (from vegetable oils, shortening and margarine) and only 10% from protein.

There is absolutely no science that proves fats and cholesterol cause cardiovascular disease, and yet we have foods that are non-fat, low fat and 2% fat, have been highly processed and contain hydrogenated fats and trans-fatty acids, the *real* hidden dangers that contribute to cancer and heart disease. The processed fats known as "trans fats" are especially dangerous. You'll see them listed on many processed foods—they're required to be mentioned on the label. These processed fats have been changed—hydrogenated—to make fully or "partially hydrogenated" trans fat. Hydrogenation is a **chemical process** in which hydrogen atoms are added to a liquid vegetable fat to change it to a *solid*—margarine being a prime example.

In Denmark, where it has been illegal for foods to contain more than 2% trans-fats since 2004, deaths from heart disease have dropped by 20%. And, in case you think I'm being overly cautious about trans fats, consider this: for each additional **2% of calories consumed as trans fat**, risk of heart disease **nearly doubles!**

Plus, trans fats not only raise total cholesterol levels, they also deplete good cholesterol (HDL), which helps protect against heart disease.

By contrast, saturated fats do NOT deplete HDL—in fact, they may even increase it!

While you don't want to overdo your fat intake, there are whole food fats I'd recommend to anyone. Start with **real butter**, which is a fat that also contains vitamin A, vitamin D, calcium, and phosphorus. Avoid the margarine-like artificial "butter" spreads out there. They are full of trans-fats and do nothing healthy for you.

Milk *can* be very healthy. However, avoid milk from conventional dairy farm operations, where cows are injected with artificial hormones to boost production. These hormones cause the cows' udders to become inflamed. This inflammation triggers white blood cells (pus) to flock to the udders. With the pus in such close proximity, you can be sure some of it will be found in the milk. Many of these cows are also milked while they are pregnant—at the very time they are producing over 30 times the estrogen as non-pregnant cows. The combined effect produces a cocktail of hormones that you may be ingesting every time you have a glass. Try **raw milk** from grass-fed cows instead. Raw milk has valuable nutrients, including conjugated linoleic acid (CLA) and lactoferrin. Lactoferrin, aside from helping the body absorb and use iron, also has strong anti-microbial and immune-enhancing abilities. If you really want a healthy milk choice consider **goat's milk**. It provides more calcium and vitamins, is less allergenic, and is more easily digested than cows milk.

Healthy Oils

Avoid cooking with hydrogenated vegetable oils, and choose one of these instead:

Coconut oil is a very stable oil (meaning it does not easily go rancid) and is excellent for use in cooking. Despite being a fat, it is even recommended in weight-loss regimens, In fact, a recent clinical study found that coconut oil reduced waistline circumference and improved cholesterol ratio. This naturally beneficial fat, rather than being bad for the heart, may actually help reduce the risk of type 2 diabetes and heart disease.

Olive oil, one of the best oils ever, reduces the risk of heart disease by lowering levels of bad LDL cholesterol and raising good HDL cholesterol levels. It is also excellent for reducing inflammation and preventing brain diseases such as Alzheimer's disease. Look for virgin or extra virgin olive oil, as it has the least amount of processing and the highest levels of beneficial compounds.

Sesame oil is another amazing oil that provides excellent taste as well as health benefits. In one study, people with high blood pressure (despite taking prescription blood pressure lowering medication) used sesame oil for cooking for 2 months and reduced their average blood pressure back to the normal range. The oil has also been found to promote weight loss, so it definitely shows that not all fats are the same.

Step 4. *Boost your fruit and veggie intake*

Fruits and vegetables are high in antioxidants, so it is absolutely critical to eat at least five servings of vegetables and two servings of fruit every day—more is even better! Be sure to choose colorful fruits and vegetables because that indicates they have high antioxidant value. There are far too many great fruits and vegetables to list them all, but here are some "super food" fruits and vegetables I absolutely recommend.

Arugula, spinach, and other greens. When it comes to greens, generally speaking the darker the color, the better. Dark leafy greens provide extra fiber, vitamins (including vitamins C and K), as well as beta-carotene. These strong antioxidants can help make sure you don't get a buildup of oxidized, bad (LDL) cholesterol.

Other dark leafy greens, including beet greens, Swiss chard, kale, and kohlrabi greens pack a powerful punch of cancer-fighting nutrients, and taste delicious sautéed with sesame oil and a little sea salt.

Sweet Potato. One of the best root vegetables around is the sweet potato. Despite the "sweet" in the name, sweet potatoes are extremely healthy, and full of fiber, beta-carotene, protein, vitamins A and C, iron and calcium. Preliminary studies have shown that sweet potatoes help balance blood sugar levels and lower insulin resistance, and are an excellent food choice for people with diabetes. However, skip the candied version with brown sugar and marshmallow topping. Instead, cut into slices and brush with olive oil, add seasoning, and either bake in the oven or grill.

Apples. The apple has been considered one of the most nutritious fruits since the Middle Ages. It was eaten to improve vision and digestion. Later, doctors insisted on its beneficial action for kidneys, the bladder and against cough and sore throat. At one point, apple cider was prescribed for kidney stone prevention. At the beginning of the 20th century, the healthy benefits of apples were somewhat forgotten by scientific researchers. In the 1970s, scientific researchers had a renewed interest for the therapeutic properties of apple. New studies are now under way for cardiovascular disease, diabetes, obesity, respiratory functions and asthma. It is known today that this fruit benefits from extraordinary nutritional, dietetic and medicinal properties.

The apple contains one of the highest concentrations of quercetin, a bioflavonoid that is a powerful antioxidant. One of the many benefits of quercetin is that it affects the glucose receptor sites and fixes on other sugar receptors as well. That means that it reduces or delays the absorption of sugar and carbohydrates, helping curb the appetite and reducing binge eating.

There is another polyphenol, called phloridzin, that is found in apples.

Like quercetin, it has similar effects on the glucose receptor sites, but it also burns fat and controls blood sugar levels.

Blueberries. Rich sources of anthocyanins and vitamin C, blueberries were ranked top in antioxidant power by researchers at Tufts University. As with most fruits and vegetables, the nutrients in blueberries support one another, working synergistically. The high anthocyanin content boosts the effects of the vitamin C in the berry, making it an immune-boosting food and helps it structurally protect blood vessels and capillaries—especially in the eyes and brain.

In fact, the ability of blueberries to protect the most delicate systems in the body is one reason why it's considered such a brain-friendly food. The combined effect of fighting oxidation in brain tissue (which left unchecked, can lead to inflammation and the formation of amyloid plaques) and supporting the tiny capillaries that supply blood to the brain has been a target of blueberry research. Consuming blueberries each day is one way to keep your focus, both literally and figuratively.

Blueberries are also an excellent source of fiber, which will keep your digestive system running smoothly and help it move processed toxins out of your body more efficiently.

Extracts of blueberries have shown strong anticancer potential, too. In one scientific study, blueberry extract inhibited TNF-alpha (an inflammatory marker) activation of JNK, a kinase involved in cell proliferation. As part of the same study, tumors in mice were decreased after being fed the blueberry extract. The researchers found that the more extract given, the smaller the tumors.

Grapes. Grapes *(Vitis vinifera)* are another easily portable fruit that makes an excellent, healthy snack. As with most fruits, the skins of grapes are loaded with valuable nutrients, including resveratrol and other health-supporting polyphenols and oligomeric proanthocyanidins (mostly known as OPCs).

OPCs are the precursor to anthocyanins—the strong antioxidants that give red, blue, and purple fruits and vegetables their antioxidant power. These powerful components protect cells from oxidative stress, and have been researched for tumor inhibition, liver detoxification, reduced blood platelet aggregation (keeping blood vessels from becoming clotted), and muscle health in athletes. In fact, in one double-blind study, the nutrients in a whole grape extract increased muscle endurance by 24%.

Aside from those kinds of immediate physical results, OPC's from grape have also been shown to have protective antioxidant effects in the brain, supporting focus and cognitive health.

A handful of raisins (dried grapes) and nuts makes a healthy and filling snack.

Pomegranate. Pomegranates *(Punica granatum)* have become popular in recent years, especially as a juice ingredient, and with good reason. Clinical and scientific research shows that this amazingly strong antioxidant supports the cardiovascular system, reduces inflammation, protects joint cartilage, and for individuals with diabetes, raises levels of glutathione (the body's own natural antioxidant) by 141%.

Although officially considered a berry, these large dark-red fruits are complex. Slice one open and you'll see a host of smaller fleshy seeds called "arils" that are rich in pomegranate juice. They can be messy, but the fruits are worth it. They are delicious tasting and provide high levels of vitamin C in addition to their already impressive levels of anthocyanins and catechins.

Like the best fruits, *everything* about the pomegranate is good for you. The bitter-tasting skin has excellent anti-inflammatory power. The seeds contain oils and fatty acids that help keep skin looking younger and modulate hormone activity, which is crucial for breast cancer prevention in women and prostate cancer prevention in men. In fact, it has been extracts of the whole fruit that have seen some of the most exciting results, showing that it inhibits prostate cancer tumor growth.

Build up your diet with fruits and vegetables

We could really spend a lot of time looking at *all* of the great benefits of fruits and vegetables. I believe that you should eat a variety each day, because they provide so many valuable nutrients. Getting the amount you need really isn't as difficult as you may think. After all, a serving of grapes is just one cup. For apples, even one small apple counts as a serving. Carrots, rich in beta-carotene and blueberries, one of my favorites, and an excellent source of anthocyanins, are just a cup per serving as well. You can easily work those foods into healthy snacks or reserve them for an energizing dessert.

STEP 5. *Eat local and organic whenever possible*

Organic food is good for you for a variety of reasons. It is grown or raised without any synthetic pesticides, insecticides, herbicides, fungicides, fertilizers or other toxic substances. Organic produce is naturally healthy—no artificial colors or flavors, and is not irradiated or genetically modified, either. Organically produced poultry, eggs, cheese, and meat are free of hormones and antibiotics. You know what you're getting—just excellent, healthful food.

Many of your local farmers may be following organic and sustainable practices, but might not have organic certification. I would suggest building a relationship with the people who provide food locally, and support their work. I think it's important to be thankful for them and your food. If you truly take an interest in your food—and I certainly encourage you to do that —consider the "farm to fork" approach: know where it's coming from, and relish the fact that it is life-building in more ways than one!

At our health food store in Green Bay, *Terry Naturally,* we host a farmers market every Wednesday and feature local "farm to fork" meals at our in-house café. It has been a huge hit. People shopping at the market make it a part of their weekly routine. Along with the excellent food, we have live music and a very family-friendly atmosphere, so it becomes a social gathering space, in addition to a great chance to buy local foods and meet friends. And isn't that what good health is all about?

STEP 6. *Avoid carbs, sugar, and processed foods*

Americans consume as much as 200 lbs of sugar a year—each! Sugar causes inflammation and is a root cause of our epidemic of obesity, heart disease and diabetes. I cannot stress enough the importance of minimizing your intake of carbohydrates and processed foods that are loaded with added, refined sugar.

Here is a Tip List of foods to avoid. Keep these foods out of your diet and you will live a longer, healthier life!

Tip #1

Avoid sugars and sweeteners

In addition to causing inflammation, sugars increase blood sugar levels, add abdominal weight, and have a terrible "crash" effect on energy levels and emotion. Because the body gains a little burst of energy from simple, readily used sugars (before the crash that triggers the next craving) many people become sugar "addicts."

Tip #2

Avoid refined flours and other grains

Refined and processed flour and other processed grains are notorious for adding to abdominal obesity, provide no real nutrition, and set up the same pattern of cravings as refined sugars and sweeteners. If you're serious about getting healthy, avoid all of them.

Tip #3
Skip refined salt

Refined salt is like any other refined food—almost everything good about it has been removed. Instead, use Celtic Sea Salt, which retains a natural multi-mineral profile.

Tip #4
Stop drinking soft drinks and fruit juice

Soft drinks are terrible. They destroy teeth at the gum line, boost blood sugar levels, and are one of the primary causes of obesity, especially in younger people. Fruit juices are hardly better. If you want the taste of fruit, eat the fruit instead. I find it incredible that fruit juices and "juice boxes" are considered the healthy alternative for children. Stay away from them!

Tip #5
Stay away from high fructose corn syrup,
artificial flavorings & colorings

High fructose corn syrup (HFCS) has been the standard sweetener for about 40 years, replacing cane sugar in many foods—even those packaged foods you wouldn't normally suspect. Just how prevalent is it? In the 20 years between 1970 and 1990, HFCS consumption increased over 1000 percent! As with artificial flavorings and colorings, it is easily avoided—just look at the labels.

Almost every processed food (and some that you wouldn't consider as "processed", like fruit juices), are sodden through with refined sugar or high-fructose corn syrup. Cut the artificial sweeteners and use stevia or a little honey if you need a touch of sweet in your diet.

Tip #6
Minimize your intake of processed foods

High in sodium, processed foods are wastelands of calories. There's nothing inherently wrong with sodium—our bodies need it for fluid, electrolyte, and pH balance. But Americans get far too much sodium in their diets. The average American **eats 40% more** than **the maximum recommended** intake for sodium—3400 mg vs. 2300 mg daily. Most of this excess sodium—about 70-75%—comes from processed foods: pizza, cured meats, soup, cold cuts, cheese, and pasta, to name a few. Too much sodium leads to fluid retention. You know that "bloated" feeling you get sometimes when you know you've had too much salty food? Unfortunately, it's doing more than just making you uncomfortable. Fluid retention increases blood volume in the body, which in turn, boosts blood pressure. The combined effect puts a lot more pressure on your kidneys to try to reach equilibrium, and of course, the increase in blood pressure makes your heart and blood vessels work a lot harder. The best thing to do is cut down on processed foods—that will reduce a lot of your excess sodium intake right away. You'll also want to add some potassium-rich foods, such as bananas or white beans, to your diet.

Tip #7
Take a pass on processed meats
Processed meats like sausage, hot dogs, deli sandwich meat and most commercial bacon is laden with nitrites, sodium, and other cancer-causing chemical preservatives. In fact, consumption of high levels of processed meat increases the risk of pancreatic cancer by 70%. The only form of bacon I would recommend is beef bacon, produced without nitrites. It can be rich in omega-3s (from grass-fed beef) and conjugated linoleic acids (CLAs), and makes a great substitute for overly processed pork bacon.

Step 7.
Plan your meals
A little planning goes a long way. You'll save time, money, and be in much better shape if you take a little time to make a healthy list, don't fall into the easy trap of relying on processed foods, and stick to healthy, easy-to-prepare whole foods.

Most Americans do not take any time to think about menu planning. Instead, they find themselves in a rush and often resort to eating out at a "fast-food" restaurant or skipping a meal. Both practices can have a negative effect on health. Take a few minutes each evening to plan the next day's menu. Or, if you can do it, plan a menu for the week. It is now easier than ever to make a meal plan using specific apps you can download for your smart phone or tablet – many of them will even generate a shopping list for you!

You'll more than recoup the time spent in planning because you'll shop more efficiently and won't find yourself missing some ingredient for the night's meal. In addition, you'll likely save money since less browsing makes it easier to avoid impulse buys.

For more on my recommendations for healthy eating, please go to my website (www.TerryTalksNutrition.com) and click on the Traditional Diet Plan. Although some people find it difficult to give up grains and sugar, once you experience the benefits of a natural way of eating (weight loss, reduced blood sugar and blood pressure levels, and increased energy) you won't have a problem eating the healthy way!

Chapter Seven

Key #7—Supplementation

Step 1
Build a strong foundation with a daily multiple

Step 2
Curcumin

Step 3
Omega-3 fatty acids

Step 4
Iodine

Step 5
Adrenal extract

Step 6
Aronia berry (black chokeberry)

Step 7
Strontium, calcium, silica and other bone-building nutrients

Step 8
Ginger

Step 9
OPCs from grape seed extract and pine bark extract

Step 10
Mesoglycan

Step 11
Boswellia

Key #7—Supplementation

Prescription drug sales in the United States are big business. The total sales for just the top ten best-selling drugs are over $150 billion dollars a year. Americans are some of the most medicated people in the world—our national average is 11.6 prescriptions per capita. West Virginia has the distinction of being the most medicated state, with a per capita average of 18.4 prescriptions.[1] What are all these drugs being used to treat? Chronic conditions such as high blood pressure, elevated cholesterol, diabetes, acid reflux and ulcers, among others. Are they effective? Are they necessary? Are they safe? In most cases I would answer **absolutely not** to all these questions. In fact, so many people die from adverse effects of prescription drugs every year that it could qualify as our fourth leading cause of death. Every year, more people die from prescription drug use or abuse than are killed in car accidents.[2]

So what is the answer to our health problems? As I outlined in Keys 5 and 6, the right kind of exercise and a proper diet can do amazing things for health. But I also believe that dietary supplements, when formulated based on solid clinical research and quality manufacturing, can treat many of the common health problems in our lives even more effectively than prescription drugs, and without the dangerous side effects. To give just one example, a combination of a high absorption curcumin with turmeric essential oils and a special extract of boswellia was shown in a clinical trial to improve mobility and reduce symptoms of knee arthritis as effectively as the prescription drug celecoxib (the generic of the brand name Celebrex®)—without **any** significant adverse effects.[3]

Why You Need Supplements

Do you know what it means to be truly healthy—mind, body and spirit? I meet thousands of people all across the county every year and I would guess that only a small percentage of them could honestly answer "yes" to this question. Most Americans have some degree of nutrient deficiency, and are so deep in their unhealthy lifestyle they don't even realize that things could be better. There is no need to be tired all the time, or get every cold that passes through the office, or suffer from chronic indigestion, sinus problems, arthritic aches and pains, or any of the other problems most people experience. The right supplements can correct nutrient deficiencies as well as treat many common problems as effectively as drugs, resulting in true, vibrant, rewarding **health**.

What to Expect from Supplements

Supplements are not magic. They cannot reverse 10 years of unhealthy living in just a week. Plan to give these products at least a three month trial before making any final decisions regarding their benefits (truthfully, many people notice a difference well before, but the best results come over time). Seek out supplement products which have proven their effectiveness in clinical trials, are formulated at therapeutic dosage levels, and are manufactured to high quality standards, and combine them with the exercise programs and diet guidelines I outlined in Keys 5 and 6. I think you will be amazed at the results.

In the following steps I will highlight the nutrients I think are most critical for establishing a foundation of good health, as well as addressing some of the problems I am asked about most often in my lectures across the country. You can also find this information on my website at www.TerryTalksNutrition.com.

STEP 1. *Build a good foundation with a daily multiple*

Let's start with what isn't needed—a once per day multivitamin. A once per day product does not contain adequate amounts of vitamins and minerals. They typically have only the RDA (Recommended Dietary Allowance) for any specific nutrient. The RDAs focus only on preventing obvious nutritional deficiencies in specific population groups. They do not define optimal intake for an individual. A tremendous amount of scientific research tells us that the RDAs can help us avoid deficiency diseases, but optimal nutrition can help us truly thrive. Additionally, vitamins are small, but minerals are huge by comparison. A once per day formula cannot contain meaningful amounts of minerals and still be of a size a person can swallow. Also not needed are artificial colors (anything labeled FD&C with a color name and number, for example: FD&C Red #40) and preservatives and other toxic ingredients (examples: corn syrup, propylene glycol, hydrogenated oils, polyvinyl alcohol, etc.)

Also unnecessary are "specialized formulas" for men, women, senior men, teen girls, etc. Looking closely at the labels of these products reveals that they are really just basic formulas with a few window dressing ingredients added—there is no real difference between them.

Humans are designed to acquire nutrients several times a day, which is why our bodies tell us to eat meals more than once per day. Water soluble vitamins are quickly flushed from the body, and should be replenished throughout the day, not just taken once in the morning or evening. That is why I consider a good foundational multivitamin one that is taken 2 or 3 times a day, has high levels of nutrients for genuine impact on health, and has the form of nutrients the body uses. Two examples of the preferred forms of nutrients are the B vitamins in their active forms, and amino-acid chelated minerals.

The B vitamins (for example, Vitamin B6, Vitamin B12 and Folate) are critical for energy, clear thinking, muscle response, exercise recovery, nervous system function and hundreds of other processes in the body.[4] Symptoms such as fatigue, anxiety, irritability, stress, forgetfulness, problems concentrating, headaches, digestive problems, and mood swings may be due to low levels of the B vitamins.[5] But did you know that the form of B vitamins used in almost all multiples has to be converted by the liver into the active forms? *And that up to 30% of the population has genetic or other problems that make them poor converters?* That is why I recommend taking B vitamins in their active forms. No conversion is necessary. Look for Vitamin B6 as pyridoxal-5-phosphate, folate as 5-methylfolate, and vitamin B12 as methylcobalamin.

Minerals are extremely important. Calcium is required to build bones and keep the heart beating properly, magnesium to regulate blood pressure, and zinc to keep the immune system strong. Other important minerals that should be in a multiple formula are chromium, molybdenum, potassium, and copper.[4]

However, minerals are difficult for the body to absorb. That is why I recommend "chelated" minerals. A "chelate" is a bond between a mineral (often called "inorganic") and an organic molecule structure, called a "ligand" that helps the body absorb the mineral during digestion. Amino acids are excellent "shepherds" of minerals through the intestinal wall, because this form can be transported directly into the cells of the body, so it can get to work right away. For example, research has shown that zinc chelated to amino acids is much better absorbed and is much more bioavailable compared to other forms of the mineral. One study comparing the absorption and bioavailability of zinc glycinate and zinc sulfate found that the glycinate form was better absorbed (51% versus 44%) and 16% more bioavailable than the sulfate (non-amino acid) form![6]

It generally does not take very long to feel the benefits of a good multivitamin. More energy, better sleep, and clearer thinking are just some of the changes you will experience. Over time, getting a good daily intake of the key vitamins and minerals I mentioned above will help reduce the risk of heart disease and cancer, increase the strength of your immune system, keep your brain alert and body strong.[7-9]

The high quality ingredients in a good multiple are not cheap. But they are absorbable and effective. What is the bigger waste of money? Spending a little more for a product that makes you feel better, or a little less money for ingredients that get flushed out of the body and down the drain without doing anything to improve health? Once you experience the benefits of taking 2 tablets, two or three times a day of a well-designed formula containing high quality ingredients, you won't be tempted by a once a day multiple again.

Step 2. *Curcumin*

If I could have only one natural medicine, it would be curcumin. This amazing compound from the turmeric root can be used to treat conditions ranging from cancer to Alzheimer's disease.[10,11] Its effectiveness is related to its ability to act as one of nature's most powerful anti-inflammatories and antioxidants. We know that almost all chronic diseases—from diabetes to arthritis to Alzheimer's disease—have something in common: unchecked, destructive inflammation. Unlike synthetic drugs, which typically work against only a single inflammation pathway, natural curcumin reduces inflammation through its effects on multiple inflammation targets, making it much more effective. Additionally, the inflammation reducing activity comes without the adverse effects associated with prescription anti-inflammatory drugs. Curcumin does not cause stomach ulcers, increase blood pressure or the risk of heart attack, destroy the liver or kidneys, or do any of the other damage associated with prescription anti-inflammatories.

Some of the most exciting new research regarding curcumin involves its use in cancer treatment. Curcumin has been shown to stop cancer initiation, promotion and progression, meaning that it stops the changes that cause normal cells to become cancerous, stops the replication of cancerous cells (tumor formation), and stops cancerous cells from migrating to other parts of the body (known as metastasis). Published studies on curcumin's anticancer activity (so far) have found that it can suppress breast, prostate, liver, skin, colon and lung cancer.[12,13]

Curcumin has also been shown to increase the activity of cancer drugs and to decrease drug resistance in cancer cells (meaning it helps cancer drugs kill tumors more efficiently). Additionally, it protects normal cells from the toxic effects of chemotherapy drugs and radiation treatments.[14] Taking curcumin in combination with chemotherapy drugs may mean less of the toxic drugs are required, but the results will be better, with significantly reduced side effects.

Researchers believe that curcumin works similarly against all types of cancer, so no matter what kind of cancer you may have, curcumin can be helpful. However, always discuss your desire to use curcumin with your cancer health professional, as there are one or two types of chemotherapy for which the benefits and specific use of curcumin has not been clarified.

Other research has shown that curcumin can reduce blood sugar levels and improve insulin response in diabetes, reduce beta amyloid levels and shrink the size of accumulated plaques by over 30% in an experimental model of Alzheimer's disease, and reduce abdominal pain and other symptoms of irritable bowel syndrome.[15-18]

There is one thing to know about curcumin, however. It is poorly absorbed (meaning that the active compounds don't easily get from the intestines into the bloodstream). That is why I recommend a curcumin that has been micronized (ground into a very fine powder) and blended with turmeric essential oil. This specialized curcumin is up to 10 times better absorbed than the standard curcumin found in most dietary supplements.[19,20] It is **as potent—or even *more* potent—at treating disease as prescription drugs**, but without the adverse effects.

I mentioned earlier that this particular form of curcumin was combined with a special extract of boswellia and shown to reduce symptoms of knee arthritis as effectively as the prescription drug celecoxib (the generic of the brand name Celebrex®). It was also used by itself by people with rheumatoid arthritis and shown to be as effective as a standard prescription drug for reducing painful, swollen, arthritic joints.[3] Of interest, 14% of the people receiving the prescription drug dropped out of the study because of adverse effects, while **no one** receiving the absorbable curcumin did so. Other clinical research that is now in progress is looking at the effectiveness of this absorbable curcumin for treating Alzheimer's disease and cancer. I think that curcumin supplementation can do as much for your health as a daily multiple, and maybe even more!

Another benefit of natural anti-inflammatories is their ability to reduce pain. I have found that combining absorbable curcumin with boswellia, nattokinase, and DLPA yields outstanding results for pain relief. Any kind of pain can be helped with these ingredients – back pain, arthritis, migraine headaches, bursitis, sprains and strains, broken bones, any kind of pain. I receive reports all the time from people with chronic pain problems who no longer need dangerous prescription medications just to get through the day, who don't need canes or walkers anymore, who finally feel good after months or years of suffering.

So to summarize, if you suffer from any inflammatory condition, or any chronic disease, the single most important supplement you can take is absorbable curcumin.

STEP 3. *Omega-3 fatty acids*

There are a few nutrients—like curcumin—that do so many amazing things that it's almost hard to believe that the stories of their benefits are true. Omega-3 fatty acids are another that fits this category. These healthy fats are not only a nutrient that you must have in your diet in order to survive (which is why they are called "essential" fatty acids), they can be helpful treatments for everything from dry skin to Alzheimer's disease.[21-23]

In fact, dry skin, along with fatigue, poor memory, poor circulation, mood swings and heart problems, are a sign of omega-3 fatty acid deficiency.

Omega-3 fatty acids, like curcumin, are natural anti-inflammatories. They are highly concentrated in the brain, which makes them very important in preventing and treating mood disorders such as depression, as well as other brain diseases such as ADD/ADHD and Alzheimer's disease. Getting enough omega-3 fatty acids during pregnancy is absolutely critical for the proper development of the fetal brain. Research has also shown that omega-3 fatty acids can reduce the symptoms of inflammatory bowel disease, decrease your risk of heart disease, heart attack and stroke, reduce your risk of cancer, and treat asthma, psoriasis, macular degeneration, and many other diseases.[24-29]

I think every person in this county could benefit from additional omega-3 fatty acids and it is another of my most frequent recommendations.

The best source of omega-3 fatty acids is cold water fish such as salmon. However, when doctors recommend additional omega-3 fatty acids, they always tell you to take fish oil. In my opinion, this is a mistake. You don't need fish oil to get omega-3 fatty acids, and using oil as a source has some negative consequences. Fish oil, especially oil that is refined and processed (as all of them are) is particularly unstable and rancid. Many of these products smell bad, will cause you to burp them back up, and need high doses—many capsules or spoons of oil—in order to be effective. The one virtue of fish oil is that you can find it everywhere. I've even seen fish oil capsules sold in gas station convenience stores.

Because of these problems, I no longer recommend fish oil as a source of omega-3 fatty acids. There is now a better way. I recommend tableted omega-3 fatty acids produced from the head of the salmon. This formula is not an oil. It is a dry tablet containing omega-3 fatty acids and phospholipids. In this form, the fatty acids are much more stable and absorbable than what is found in the old fish oil products where the fatty acids are bound to triglycerides. They can be extracted using just water and enzymes, and don't require the heat, processing and solvents used to produce fish oils. Because these phospholipid fatty acids are so stable, they don't get rancid, taste bad, or give you fish burps. Just one or two tablets a day of phospholipid omega-3 is all you need to keep your body healthy.

STEP 4. *Iodine*

Once one of the most commonly used medicines in the world, iodine was "forgotten" in favor of new pharmaceutical drugs. However, this misunderstood mineral is still one of the most powerful natural medicines available, and is probably my second most frequent recommendation after curcumin. Without iodine, the thyroid gland cannot function—iodine (along with the amino acid, l-tyrosine) is required to create thyroid hormones. Additionally, iodine detoxifies dangerous, cancer-causing toxic elements such as fluoride, bromide and chloride.[30,31] It is very effective at reducing the risk of cancer, especially breast cancer. Iodine can also be used to treat other breast diseases, such as the painful condition, fibrocystic breast disease. In fact, in one study, 98% of women with fibrocystic breast disease receiving iodine treatment were pain-free by the study's end, and 72% had improvements in breast tissue.[32] I recommend iodine supplementation for anyone with low thyroid function (hair loss, weight gain, constantly cold, fatigue, dry skin, mood changes, etc.) and as part of a cancer treatment plan, especially breast cancer. For more about iodine I suggest reading the book *Iodine: Why You Need It, Why You Can't Live Without It,* by Dr. David Brownstein.

Different body tissues prefer iodine in different forms, which is why I recommend supplementing with iodine as a combination of potassium iodide, sodium iodide and molecular iodine. Thyroid tissue absorbs iodine as potassium iodide, while breast and prostate tissue have a greater affinity for iodine as molecular iodide.[33] For targeted treatment of low thyroid function, I recommend taking a combination of the three types of iodine with the amino acid l-tyrosine to best increase thyroid hormone levels and thyroid function.

One of the biggest controversies surrounding iodine is how much is needed. The RDA (remember, this is the minimum amount needed to prevent symptoms of nutrient deficiency) in adults is only 150 micrograms. Holistic medicine practitioners routinely recommend much higher amounts to treat hypothyroidism, cancer, and other diseases. A typical maintenance dosage for an adult would be 12.5 mgs (12,500 micrograms). In certain cases, or to saturate the body with iodine, 50 mgs per day is recommended. For breast cancer, possibly 100 mg of iodine per day is appropriate, although I would urge you to discuss this with your integrative practitioner. For more information on the benefits of iodine, especially for low thyroid function, please go to my website at www.TerryTalksNutrition.com to find some excellent articles on this topic.

STEP 5. *Adrenal extract*

Adrenal gland problems are often mistaken for thyroid gland problems. The adrenal glands secrete hormones (such as cortisol) that allow the body to cope with stress. However, in situations of chronic stress, the adrenal glands can become depleted and not function efficiently.[34] Signs of adrenal burnout include: falling asleep at night, but waking up again at midnight or later, craving salt or sugar, exhaustion after exercising, feeling overwhelmed or even filled with dread. Other symptoms which may occur are sensitivity to cold, hypotension, weak cardiac action and pulse, anorexia, slow metabolism, and constipation. People with adrenal insufficiency usually have many symptoms associated with upper respiratory problems. They are the ones who always have a cold, allergies, hives and usually anything that goes around.

I highly recommend the use of bovine adrenal gland extract to address adrenal fatigue and burnout. Adrenal gland extract contains natural hormones and nutrients that are used by the adrenal glands in returning them to proper function. Additionally, B vitamins are necessary, particularly vitamin B6 (as P5P, the biologically active form of B6) and pantothenic acid. L-tyrosine is required to produce the adrenal gland hormones epinephrine and norepinephrine. The only place in the body that vitamin C is temporarily stored is in the adrenal glands. DHEA and pregnenolone are two adrenal hormones that are precursors for all other hormones. There are also two herbs that I would heavily rely on to support adrenal function: licorice root extract *(Glycyrrhiza glabra)* and Rehmannia *(Rehmannia glutinosa)*. Both support liver function, help prevent adrenal hormones from prematurely breaking down, and aid in a normal response to daily stress.[35-45]

Another excellent way to restore adrenal gland function is with adaptogens. Adaptogens are herbs that bring balance to the body. They are especially useful when dealing with the physical signs of stress. By increasing energy, relieving anxiety, strengthening the immune system, and improving focus and concentration, the adaptogenic herbs can make a real difference to quality of life. I recommend two traditional adaptogens: rhodiola, and ashwaghanda. These herbs affect adrenal gland function through their ability to influence the HPA (hypothalamic-pituitary-adrenal) axis, a part of the body's stress response system, and have been shown in clinical studies to increase energy and mental concentration.[46-58]

Properly supporting the adrenal glands, as well as addressing any underlying thyroid issues, can make a significant difference of your overall health.

STEP 6. *Aronia berry (black chokeberry)*

Berries, including blueberry, strawberry, and cranberry, are all well known for their health benefits and I frequently recommend them, both as foods and in supplements. However, if there is one berry that stands out from the rest, it is aronia, or black chokeberry. Aronia is one of the richest natural sources of anythocyanins, the plant compounds which give fruits and berries their rich red, blue and purple color. However, anthocyanins don't just add color—they also do amazing things for health. Just a few of their benefits include: reducing blood pressure, boosting the immune system, protecting the liver, improving vision, reducing inflammation, and suppressing the spread of cancer cells.[59]

Fresh aronia berries are very tart and not everyone enjoys them. However, a clinically studied aronia extract is also available as a supplement. There is a wide range of research on supplemental aronia, including its benefits in cancer patients.

Aronia is a very powerful antioxidant, meaning that it neutralizes unstable molecules called free radicals. Free radical activity is a known risk factor for cancer, but what many people don't know is that conventional cancer therapy—chemotherapy and radiation therapy—also increases the number of free radicals (or oxidative stress). Free radical activity during cancer treatment can also increase the risk of side effects such as fatigue or blood clots. In a clinical study, administration of an aronia extract significantly reduced free radical levels and oxidative stress in patients receiving surgery and chemotherapy for breast cancer.[60]

In an experimental model, aronia protected against the adverse effects of smoking. Other research has found that aronia reduces inflammation, normalizes carbohydrate metabolism in experimental models of diabetes, suppresses cancer cell growth and has antiviral activity against the flu virus.[61,62] While I encourage everyone to get plenty of fresh fruit in their diet, if you are looking for a powerful antioxidant supplement with a wide range of benefits, there is no better recommendation I can make than aronia.

STEP 7. *Strontium, calcium, silica and other bone-building nutrients*

When you think about bone density and preventing osteoporosis (brittle bones) you probably assume it is just a matter of getting more calcium. While it is true that calcium is an important part of the bone building process, it is not the whole story. When considering calcium, **quantity is not as important as the quality.** For example, calcium citrate is 2.5 times more bioavailable than calcium carbonate.[63]

Also, less calcium is needed when it is combined with many of the accessory nutrients that help provide better calcium absorption. I like to recommend a moderate level of calcium as calcium citrate and calcium malate, in the 400-600 mg range per day instead of the excessive 1,000-1,500 mg as advised by some nutritionists. Too high a calcium intake can suppress the essential vitamin D circulating in our bloodstream. Vitamin D is crucial in maintaining healthy bones, (and cellular health overall), so by overdoing it with *too much* calcium, you may actually undermine the natural process of bone building in the body.

In addition to calcium and vitamin D (at least 4,000 IU daily) some of the other nutrients that I consider crucial for daily use to increase bone density are magnesium, zinc, copper, manganese, fructoborate (boron), silicon, vitamin K1 and K2, and the beneficial probiotic, *Lactobacillus sporogenes.* Each of these has a unique role in supporting bone metabolism. For example, fructoborate is a special form of boron from plants, naturally combined with other stable compounds that help boron target the tissues that need it most. Fructoborate has been clinically shown to reduce joint pain in individuals suffering from mild to moderate osteoarthritis. Plus, fructoborate helps the body absorb vitamin D much more efficiently as well. Vitamin K2, also called menaquinone, is extracted from the Japanese fermented food, natto. This unique form of vitamin K has special properties beyond that of traditional vitamin K. This very effective vitamin is essential for the body to utilize calcium to build healthy bone tissue. It activates osteocalcin, a protein required to bind calcium to the mineral matrix and strengthen bones. These are just two examples of the unique ways the nutrients I recommend increase bone density and prevent bone disease such as osteoporosis.[64-82]

One mineral I think is extremely important for bones is **strontium.** Strontium can have a tremendous effect in positively changing bone health and bone density. In fact, it can fight and possibly even *reverse* osteoporosis. A three year randomized, double-blind, placebo controlled study of strontium for bone density (published in the *New England Journal of Medicine*) revealed that women suffering from osteoporosis and treated with strontium experienced a 41% reduction in risk of a vertebral fracture compared to the placebo group. Overall vertebrae (bones that make up the spinal column) density in the strontium group increased 6.8% but there was a 1.3% decrease in the placebo group. Other studies have found similar benefits.[83-86]

It is important to know that strontium and calcium fight for the same absorption pathway in the body, and strontium will always win. Therefore, take your calcium and strontium supplements at least 2 hours apart. I would suggest taking 680 mg of strontium once a day.

Another exciting supplement for bone support is **silica**. Silica is a crucial trace mineral found in bones and fast growing tissues like hair, skin, and fingernails. It's also a major building block of collagen, which helps keep skin supple and blood vessels strong, as well as to make strong bones. Lack of silica in the diet causes defects in collagen and skeletal bone. However, increasing silica intake through supplements can dramatically increase bone density. A specific silica extract from horsetail has been shown to have an amazing ability to increase calcium absorption into bone by over 50%, increase the formation of collagen and speed healing of bone fractures. A randomized, double blind, placebo controlled study of 65 women over 12 months revealed that this special silica extract from horsetail, blended with marine oils, reduced bone destruction and increased bone strength. Another study was performed on 150 individuals with varying degrees of bone fracture. Doctors reported that in 80% of participants, significant improvements in bone healing were evident after 15 days of use, and further gains were measurable after 6 weeks of use.[87-90]

Another use for this special silica is dental implants. Implants in the jaw bone are commonly used for crowns, bridges and dentures, as well as for other treatments. In clinical use, dentists reported that, when patients took the special silica extract, implants integrated into bone tissue 50% faster—without pain and inflammation.[91]

One of the keys to the great results obtained with this special silica is a unique soluble water extraction process (no chemicals, no solvents) that preserves the silica's natural bond to companion compounds (flavonoids) from horsetail, while filtering out the insoluble parts, which are abrasive and harmful if ingested. After this purification and extraction, the compounds are micronized (very small particles) and blended with marine lipids.

Marine lipids are **nature's perfect transport mechanism** for absorption and utilization within the body. It does not matter how much silica you ingest—what matters is how much is absorbed, and the small particle size and marine lipids ensure a very absorbable, effective form of silica.

The best way to prevent bone disease is to build strong bones early in your life. However, it is *never* too late to take better care of your bones. Calcium with the other key vitamins and minerals mentioned above, including strontium and silica, can not only prevent, but can also reverse, excessive bone loss.

Step 8. *Ginger*

Like curcumin, ginger is a natural spice and a potent natural medicine. It is well known as a digestive aid able to calm an upset stomach, in addition to being a potent anti-inflammatory. Most ginger products are extracts made from the dried and powdered ginger root.

Ginger is useful for all types of indigestion—morning sickness, motion sickness, nausea, upset stomach, gas and diarrhea. New research has found that ginger can help reduce nausea and vomiting induced by cancer treatments, specifically radiation therapy. In fact, one interesting study found that ginger taken during radiation therapy protected normal cells from damaging radiation, so that only the dangerous tumor cells were destroyed.[92] Ginger has also been shown to reduce nausea associated with cancer chemotherapy drugs. This side effect is extremely common, with over 70% of patients receiving chemotherapy reporting they have experienced nausea. In fact, ginger has been reported to reduce cancer-treatment associated nausea as effectively as a prescription anti-nausea drug.[93-94]

One of ginger's best known benefits is its ability to minimize nausea associated with motion sickness. In some very well-known studies, otherwise healthy people were seated in a spinning chair, or in the new research seated in a drum whose striped sides rotated around the chair instead, until they reported feeling nauseous. When the volunteers received ginger before they experienced motion, the time to feeling nauseous was longer, and the degree of nausea they experienced was less.[95-96]

Nausea and vomiting in pregnancy is extremely common—up to 90% of women experience these symptoms in their first trimester of pregnancy.[97]

Ginger can safely and effectively relieve pregnancy-associated nausea and morning sickness, and can even work as effectively as prescription anti-nausea medications. Ginger has been administered in a variety of dosage levels and formats, but 1 gram of ginger daily is a suggested dose.[98-99] Some expert sources caution against the use of ginger in pregnancy, despite the fact that no clinical evidence has ever found it harmful. However, because pregnancy is a very sensitive time, it is important to always discuss use of any dietary supplements with your healthcare provider.

Finally, ginger is excellent for reducing inflammation. Ginger works both on reducing muscle pain caused by exercise and physical exertion, as well as in relieving pain and inflammation associated with chronic conditions such as arthritis.[100-101] I like to combine ginger with curcumin, boswellia and DLPA for superior relief of pain.

Although these are the better known health benefits of ginger, it can also be helpful as an antioxidant to reduce oxidative stress levels, relieve migraine headache pain, boost immune system activity, improve cholesterol levels, and enhance circulation and heart function. In short, ginger is an herb with many significant benefits and almost everyone can feel better by adding ginger to their supplement regimen.[102]

Step 9. *OPCs from grape seed extract and pine bark extract*

You may be familiar with the "French paradox"—the observation that despite the traditional French diet, which is high in cholesterol and saturated fats, the French have unexpectedly low levels of heart disease. One explanation for this is that the French also consume plentiful amounts of red grapes and red wine. While grapes and red wine do contain very healthy compounds, some of the most significant benefits in grapes are from a part of the fruit avoided by most Americans—the seeds. Grape seeds are a source of oligomeric proanthocyandins, or OPCs. These natural antioxidants, also found in pine bark extract, are able to neutralize dangerous free radicals that can damage tiny blood vessels, increasing your risk of heart attack or stroke. Research has also found that they can protect against cancer and diabetes, reduce inflammation, improve memory, and even help prevent weight gain![103-107]

While I do not agree that cholesterol is dangerous and that high cholesterol levels cause heart disease, I do think that preventing the oxidation of LDL cholesterol is an important step in reducing your risk of heart attack or stroke. Oxidized LDL cholesterol in the blood stream can damage the walls of the arteries, trigger inflammation, and lead to a build-up of cholesterol, white blood cells, and other fats to form a plaque. Plaques can block blood flow, or rupture and cause a heart attack.

OPCs, because of their antioxidant properties, are excellent for preventing LDL cholesterol from oxidizing. In a study of OPCs from pine bark, accumulation of oxidized LDL in the arteries was reduced by 38%! A separate study of pine bark extract found that it increased HDL (beneficial) cholesterol levels. Even a 1% increase in HDL can have a 2-3% decrease in heart attack risk, so anything that increases HDL while also preventing the oxidation of LDL can significantly reduce your risk of heart disease.[108]

OPCs are also helpful for other problems with arteries, veins and circulation, including chronic venous insufficiency (CVI). In a clinical study of pine bark extract in patients with CVI, researchers reported use of the extract was associated with reduced leg swelling and heaviness. A random-ized, double-blind trial of pine bark extract also found that it was able to reduce blood pressure levels.[109-111]

One of the most interesting benefits of OPCs is the ability to prevent weight gain. Obesity is strongly associated with inflammation, so it is no surprise that the anti-inflammatory activity of grape seed and pine bark extracts is helpful to counter weight gain. However, OPCs have also been found to inhibit fat-metabolizing enzymes, leading to less fat absorption and less fat accumulation in the body's fat cells. Additionally, OPCs help increase sensitivity to insulin, thus reducing insulin resistance, one of the hallmark signs of metabolic syndrome, diabetes, and obesity.[112-115]

While I think that grape seed and pine bark extracts are very beneficial supplements, choosing a product is critical to getting good results. Whether the extract is high in beneficial compounds or full of useless tannins, it can still legally be labeled as "grape seed extract" or "pine bark extract." There-fore, make sure the product you purchase is pure and high in monomers, dimers and trimers, and guaranteed *free of tannins*. Unfortunately, there are plenty of cheap products containing only tannins on the market. These are a waste of your money. Tannins are not absorbed in the intestines and, in fact, may be harmful to your health. Avoid them and look for quality products standardized for OPC levels.

STEP 10. *Mesoglycan*

One in every three deaths in America is due to heart disease or stroke—equivalent to 2,200 deaths every day. Heart disease is also expensive—over $400 billion dollars a year in healthcare costs and lost productivity. Totaling high blood pressure, oxidized LDL cholesterol and atherosclerosis, chronic inflammation, and even other diseases such as diabetes and abnormal thyroid levels are associated with developing heart disease. In the steps above, I have highlighted a few very effective natural medicines which can significantly reduce the risk of heart problems, including curcumin, omega-3 fatty acids, aronia, and grape seed and pine bark extracts.[116]

However, there is one more ingredient I want to mention that is truly outstanding at preventing heart disease and treating problems with veins and arteries. Mesoglycan (also known as glycosaminoglycans or mucopolysaccharide) has been shown to prevent or slow atherosclerosis (hardening of the arteries) as well as to treat other vascular diseases, including varicose veins and hemorrhoids. Mesoglycan has more than one mechanism of action. Most importantly, it works on the actual formation of the blood vessel walls, aiding them to be strong, yet flexible. Additionally, mesoglycan uniquely helps improve blood flow and circulation by decreasing the concentration of compounds associated with clotting (fibrinogen) *without* adversely affecting the normal and necessary process of blood coagulation.[117-118]

In clinical studies, mesoglycan has been shown to help vessel walls remain flexible, as well as to decrease plasma fibrinogen (reducing the risk of abnormal clotting) in patients who had previously suffered a stroke. It has also been shown to increase the ability to walk without pain in patients with intermittent claudication (a disease in which poor blood flow during movement or exercise causes pain and cramping in the legs) as well as reduce pain and swelling associated with deep vein thrombosis and chronic venous insufficiency. A venous skin ulcer is a shallow wound that forms when blood pools, usually in the legs, instead of being pushed back to the heart. In patients with this problem who were treated with mesoglycan, the ulcers healed faster and more completely versus patients receiving a placebo treatment. In a small clinical study of patients with diabetes who also suffered from diabetic retinopathy—damage to the small blood vessels in the back of the eyes—mesoglycan administration was associated with reduced levels of tears and damage to these small and delicate blood vessels and improvement in blood flow. No patients in the placebo group experienced any improvement.[119-123]

These are just a few of the many clinical reports on the benefits of mesoglycan. In summary, mesoglycan helps build strong and flexible blood vessels, as well as improve blood flow to the heart. I recommend it for any problem involving veins and circulation: atherosclerosis, varicose veins, hemorrhoids, chronic venous insufficiency, diabetic retinopathy, etc. When you choose a mesoglycan product make sure to select one that is standardized for its key compounds (such as heparan sulfate) and is the clinically studied formula.

STEP 11. *Boswellia*

It is difficult to pick just a few key areas to build a foundation plan for good health. I recommend many different ingredients and formulas every day, and I'm always learning about exciting new research and nutrients. However, I realized there is one final recommendation that can benefit so many people that I could not possibly leave it off my list in this book.

Boswellia (also known as frankincense) is a close second to curcumin for my favorite herbal medicine. It has been a part of traditional medicine in India, called Ayurveda, for thousands of years, and was used by Ayurvedic practitioners for the treatment of arthritis, coughs, asthma, ulcerative colitis, sores, and even snakebite. One of the interesting things I learned about the use of boswellia is that in India it is considered a natural disinfectant, and is burned to help control bacteria. This natural antibacterial activity also explains why boswellia is helpful at healing wounds and sores.

Like curcumin, boswellia is a powerful natural anti-inflammatory. Research has shown that the boswellic acids—the active compounds in boswellia—inhibit the activity of the 5-LOX enzyme, which leads to decreased levels of inflammatory compounds called leukotrienes. Because of its effects in reducing 5-LOX activity and leukotriene levels, boswellia is excellent for treating inflammatory conditions of the lungs and intestines (which are associated with the 5-LOX inflammatory pathway) such as asthma, COPD, inflammatory bowel and Crohn's disease. Boswellia is also an excellent partner for curcumin, and as I mentioned above, a special combination of curcumin and boswellia was shown in a clinical trial to improve mobility and reduce inflammation associated with arthritis of the knee as effectively as the prescription drug celecoxib (the generic of the brand name Celebrex®)—without any significant adverse effects. It has also been shown to reduce joint pain and stiffness associated with rheumatoid arthritis.[124] And finally, new research has shown that boswellia has anti-cancer activity, and may help prevent the growth and spread of cancer cells, especially colon cancer, and brain tumors.[125,126]

To get the best benefits from boswellia, I recommend extracts which have at least 10% AKBA, one of the key inflammation reducing compounds in boswellia, and less than 5% of beta boswellic acids. The beta boswellic acids can actually reduce boswellia's inflammation fighting activity, which is why reducing them to less than 5% makes the boswellia extract up to 10 times more potent.

Boswellia is one of the most powerful medicines found in nature. Taken alone, or in combination with curcumin and other natural ingredients, I recommend it for any disease that involves chronic inflammation as well as for overall health and prevention of cancer.

Get the most from your natural supplements

If you wish to achieve optimum results with natural supplements, you must remember that they are not the same as drugs. The field of natural medicine provides an entirely different approach to building and maintaining great health.

Drugs are designed to mask symptoms, often providing immediate relief but failing to achieve the long-lasting benefits that can be gained through natural supplements.

Natural products do not mask symptoms. Instead, they target the source of your body's needs and deliver the long-lasting benefits you're really looking for. Sometimes these benefits are achieved relatively quickly...and sometimes they take a little time. I urge you to use all natural products for the recommended length of time. It is also very important that you use them consistently. In other words, don't skip a day here and a day there. If you use quality natural products as recommended, you will get results.

Shop to live at your local health food store

Because quality is so vital to the efficacy of natural products, your best resource for dependable products and reliable information is your neighborhood health food store. There, you'll find experts and expertise, and can talk to a knowledgeable person who understands more about natural products than a part-time stocker in a supermarket.

Neighborhood health food stores are in the business of promoting health. To this end, most sell top-quality products and know their vendors well. Store owners usually stand behind the products they sell and many offer money-back guarantees.

You'll find lots of great educational materials at most health food stores. Many offer racks of the latest books and scientific pamphlets. Local stores also offer seminars and guest speakers throughout the year.

The information I've just shared with you may seem a bit overwhelming. Yet I believe that the more you understand natural products, the better chance you have of making intelligent choices. An informed person gets the most value for his or her money.

Choosing natural products isn't like picking out a shampoo or a garden hose or a car. You can replace your car, but you can't replace the human body. When you purchase natural products, you're making these choices for your most precious possession—your health. By choosing high-quality nutritional and herbal supplements and natural medicines, you're investing in your most valuable resource.

Final Thoughts

The ideas and philosophies I have outlined in this short book have been the foundation for the success I have attained in my life—including physical, mental and spiritual health. I hope that you have been inspired by these pages to make lasting changes in your own life so that you can experience true vibrant health for yourself. I always welcome your comments and questions, whether you need advice on natural supplements or an encouraging word on your own journey to health.

Please feel free to contact me with your comments or questions. For more information, go to my website at **www.TerryTalksNutrition.com.** I look forward to hearing from you!

Chapter 7 References

1. The Most Medicated States. Available at: http://www.forbes.com/2010/08/16/ medications-pharmaceuticals-drugs-medicine-lifestyle-health-rx.html. Accessed on December 27, 2012.

2. Reinberg S. Drug Overdoses Kill More Americans Than Car Accidents: CDC. Available at: http://healthfinder.gov/news/newsstory.aspx?docID=660008. Accessed on December 18, 2012.

3. Antony B, Kizhakedath R, Benny M, Kuruvilla BT. Clinical Evaluation of a herbal product in the management of knee osteoarthritis. Abstract 316. *Osteoarthritis Cartilage.* 2011;19(S1):S145-S146.

4. Hendler SS. PDR for *Nutritional Supplements*, 2nd ed. Physicians' Desk Reference, Inc. Montvale, NJ; 2008.

5. Combs GF, Jr. *The Vitamins: Fundamental Aspects in Nutrition and Health.* Academic Press, Inc. San Diego, CA; 1992.

6. Schlegel P, Windisch W. Bioavailability of zinc glycinate in comparison with zinc sulphate in the presence of dietary phytate in an animal model with Zn labelled rats. *J Anim Physiol Anim Nutr* (Berl). 2006 Jun;90(5-6):216-22.

7. Gaziano JM; Sesso HD, Christen WG, et al. Multivitamins in the prevention of cancer in men: the Physicians' Health Study II randomized controlled trial. *JAMA.* 2012 Nov 14;308(18):1871-80.

8. Rautiainen S, Akesson A, Levitan EB, et al. Multivitamin use and the risk of myocardial infarction: a population-based cohort of Swedish women. *Am J Clin Nutr.* 2010 Nov;92(5):1251-6. doi: 10.3945/ajcn.2010.29371.

9. Grima NA, Pase MP, Macpherson H, Pipingas A. The effects of multivitamins on cognitive performance: a systematic review and meta-analysis. *J Alzheimers Dis.* 2012;29(3):561-9.

10. Goel A, Jhurani S, Aggarwal BB. Multi-targeted therapy by curcumin: how spicy is it? *Mol Nutr Food Res.* 2008;52(9):1010-30.

11. Aggarwal BB, Sundaram C, Malani N, Ichikawa H. Curcumin: the Indian solid gold. *Adv Exp Med Biol.* 2007;595:1-75.

12. Shehzad A, Wahid F, Lee YS. Curcumin in cancer chemoprevention: molecular targets, pharmacokinetics, bioavailability, and clinical trials. *Arch Pharm (Weinheim).* 2010;343(9):489-99.

13. Johnson JJ, Mukhtar H. Curcumin for chemoprevention of colon cancer. *Cancer Lett.* 2007;255(2):170-81.

14. Goel A, Aggarwal BB. Curcumin, the golden spice from Indian saffron, is a chemosensitizer and radiosensitizer for tumors and chemoprotector and radioprotector for normal organs. *Nutr Cancer.* 2010;62(7):919-30.

15. Na LX, Zhang YL, Li Y, et al. Curcumin improves insulin resistance in skeletal muscle of rats. *Nutr Metab Cardiovasc Dis.* 2011 Jul;21(7):526-33.

16. Seo KI, Choi MS, Jung UJ, et al. Effect of curcumin supplementation on blood glucose, plasma insulin, and glucose homeostasis related enzyme activities in diabetic db/db mice. *Mol Nutr Food Res.* 2008;52(9):995-1004.

17. Garcia-Alloza M. Curcumin labels amyloid pathology in vivo, disrupts existing plaques, and partially restores distorted neurites in an Alzheimer mouse model. *J Neurochem.* 2007;102:1095-1104.

18. Bundy R, Walker AF, Middleton RW, Booth J. Turmeric extract may improve irritable bowel syndrome symptomology in otherwise healthy adults: a pilot study. *J Altern Complement Med.* 2004;10(6):1015-8.

19. Antony B, Merina B, Iyer VS, et al. A pilot cross-over study to evaluate human oral bioavailability of BCM-95CG (Biocurcumax), a novel bioenhanced preparation of curcumin. *Indian J Pharm Sci.* 2008;70(4):445-449.

20. Benny M, Antony B. Bioavailability of BioCurcumax™ (BCM-095™). *Spice India.* September, 2006 :11-15.

21. Lin PY, Chiu CC, Huang SY, Su KP. A meta-analytic review of polyunsaturated fatty acid compositions in dementia. *J Clin Psychiatry.* 2012;73(9):1245-54.

22. Russell FD, Bürgin-Maunder CS. Distinguishing health benefits of eicosapentaenoic and docosahexaenoic acids. *Mar Drugs.* 2012;10(11):2535-59.

23. Gerber M. Omega-3 fatty acids and cancers: a systematic update review of epidemiological studies. *Br J Nutr.* 2012;107 Suppl 2:S228-39.

24. Fleith M, Clandinin MT. Dietary PUFA for preterm and term infants: review of clinical studies. *Crit Rev Food Sci Nutr.* 2005;45(3):205-29.

25. McCusker MM, Grant-Kels JM. Healing fats of the skin: the structural and immunologic roles of the omega-6 and omega-3 fatty acids. *Clin Dermatol.* 2010;28(4):440-51.

26. Mori TA, Beilin LJ. Omega-3 fatty acids and inflammation. *Curr Atheroscler Rep.* 2004;6(6):461-7.

27. Siriwardhana N, Kalupahana NS, Moustaid-Moussa N. Health benefits of n-3 polyunsaturated fatty acids: eicosapentaenoic acid and docosahexaenoic acid. *Adv Food Nutr Res.* 2012;65:211-22.

28. Simopoulos AP. Omega-3 fatty acids in inflammation and autoimmune diseases. *J Am Coll Nutr.* 2002;21(6):495-505.

29. Calder PC. The role of marine omega-3 (n-3) fatty acids in inflammatory processes, atherosclerosis and plaque stability. *Mol Nutr Food Res.* 2012;56(7):1073-80.

30. Rheault S. Iodine: functions and benefits beyond the thyroid. Townsend Letter. 2008 (December).

31. Wright JV. The "medicine cabinet" mineral that's a surprising breast health hero. *Nutrition and Healing.* 2012:19(7):1-3,6-8.

32. Ghent WR, et al. Iodine replacement in fibrocystic disease of the breast. *Can J Surg* 1993;36:453-460.

33. Reinhardt W, Kohl S, Hollmann D, Klapp G, Benker G, Reinwein D, Mann K. Efficacy and safety of iodine in the postpartum period in an area of mild iodine deficiency. *Eur J Med Res.* 1998;3(4):203-10.

34. Teitelbaum J. Chapter 6: Hormonal Imbalances. In: *Real Cause Real Cure: the 9 root causes of the most common health problems and how to solve them.* Rodale Books. 2012.

35. Padayatty SJ, Doppman JL, Chang R, Human adrenal glands secrete vitamin C in response to adrenocorticotrophic hormone. *Am J Clin Nutr.* 2007;86(1):145-9.

36. Allolio B, Arlt W, Hahner S. DHEA: why, when, and how much—DHEA replacement in adrenal insufficiency. *Ann Endocrinol* (Paris). 2007;68(4):268-73.

37. Johannsson G, Burman P, Wirén L, et al. Low dose dehydroepiandrosterone affects behavior in hypopituitary androgen-deficient women: a placebo-controlled trial. *J Clin Endocrinol Metab.* 2002;87(5):2046-52.

38. Binder G, Weber S, Ehrismann M, et al. Effects of dehydroepiandrosterone therapy on pubic hair growth and psychological well-being in adolescent girls and young women with central adrenal insufficiency: a double-blind, randomized, placebo-controlled phase III trial. *J Clin Endocrinol Metab.* 2009;94(4):1182-90.

39. Deijen JB, Orlebeke JF. Effect of tyrosine on cognitive function and blood pressure under stress. *Brain Res Bull.* 1994;33(3):319-23

40. Isbrucker RA, Burdock GA. Risk and safety assessment on the consumption of Licorice root (Glycyrrhiza sp.), its extract and powder as a food ingredient, with emphasis on the pharmacology and toxicology of glycyrrhizin. *Regul Toxicol Pharmacol.* 2006c;46(3):167-92.

41. Soucy P, Luu-The V. Conversion of pregnenolone to DHEA by human 17alpha-hydroxylase/17, 20-lyase (P450c17). Evidence that DHEA is produced from the released intermediate, 17alpha-hydroxypregnenolone. *Eur J Biochem.* 2000;267(11):3243-7

42. Glandulars. In: Hendler SS, ed. *PDR for Nutritional Supplements.* 2nd ed. Montvale, NJ: Physician's Desk Reference; 2008:264.

43. Vitamin B6. In: In: Hendler SS, ed. PDR for *Nutritional Supplements.* 2nd ed. Montvale, NJ: Physician's Desk Reference; 2008:634-644

44. Coombs G. Pantothenic Acid. In: *The Vitamins: Fundamental Aspects in Nutrition and Health.* San Diego, California: Academic Press, Inc; 1992:345-356.

45. Dharmananda S. Rehmannia. Available at: http://www.itmonline.org/arts/rehmann. htm. Accessed on December 27, 2012.

46. Olsson EM, von Schéele B, Panossian AG. A randomised, double-blind, placebo-controlled, parallel-group study of the standardised extract shr-5 of the roots of Rhodiola rosea in the treatment of subjects with stress-related fatigue. *Planta* Med. 2009;75(2):105-12.

47. 2. Darbinyan V, Kteyan A, Panossian A, Gabrielian E, Wikman G, Wagner H. Rhodiola rosea in stress induced fatigue—a double blind cross-over study of a standardized extract SHR-5 with a repeated low-dose regimen on the mental performance of healthy physicians during night duty. *Phytomedicine.* 2000;7(5):365-71.

48. 3. Spasov AA, Wikman GK, Mandrikov VB, Mironova IA, Neumoin VV. A double-blind, placebo-controlled pilot study of the stimulating and adaptogenic effect of Rhodiola rosea SHR-5 extract on the fatigue of students caused by stress during an examination period with a repeated low-dose regimen. *Phytomedicine.* 2000;7(2):85-9.

49. 4. Cicero AF, Derosa G, Brillante R, Bernardi R, Nascetti S, Gaddi A. Effects of Siberian ginseng (Eleutherococcus senticosus maxim.) on elderly quality of life: a randomized clinical trial. *Arch Gerontol Geriatr Suppl.* 2004;(9):69-73

50. 5. Asano K, Takahashi T, Miyashita M, et al. Effect of Eleuteroccocus senticosus Extract on Human Physical Working Capacity. *Planta* Med. 1986;52(3):175-7

51. 6. Kimura Y, Sumiyoshi M. Effects of various Eleutherococcus senticosus cortex on swimming time, natural killer activity and corticosterone level in forced swimming stressed mice. *J Ethnopharmacol.* 2004;95(2-3):447-53.

52. 7. Bhattacharya SK, Muruganandam AV. Adaptogenic activity of Withania somnifera: an experimental study using a rat model of chronic stress. *Pharmacol Biochem Behav.* 2003;75(3):547-55.

53. 8. Singh A, Naidu PS, Gupta S, Kulkarni SK. Effect of natural and synthetic antioxidants in a mouse model of chronic fatigue syndrome. *J Med Food.* 2002;5(4):211-20

54. 9. Mahdi AA, Shukla KK, Ahmad MK, et al. Withania somnifera improves semen quality in stress-related male fertility. *Evid Based Complement Alternat Med.* 2009.

55. 10. Ahmad MK, Mahdi AA, Shukla KK, et al. Withania somnifera improves semen quality by regulating reproductive hormone levels and oxidative stress in seminal plasma of infertile males. *Fertil Steril.* 2009.

56. 11. Sun LJ, Wang GH, Wu B, et al. Effects of schisandra on the function of the pituitary-adrenal cortex, gonadal axis and carbohydrate metabolism in rats undergoing experimental chronic psychological stress, navigation and strenuous exercise. *Zhonghua Nan Ke Xue.* 2009;15(2):126-9.

57. 12. Panossian A, Wikman G. Pharmacology of Schisandra chinensis Bail.: an overview of Russian research and uses in medicine. *J Ethnopharmacol.* 2008;118(2):183-212.

58. 13. Guo LY, Hung TM, Bae KH, et al. Anti-inflammatory effects of schisandrin isolated from the fruit of Schisandra chinensis Baill. *Eur J Pharmacol.* 2008;591(1-3):293-9

59. Konczek I, Zhang W. Anthocyanins: more than Nature's colors. *J Biomed Biotechnol.* 2004; 2004(5): 239–240.

60. Kedzierska M, Malinowska J, Kontek B, et al. Chemotherapy modulates the biological activity of breast cancer patients plasma: the protective properties of black chokeberry extract. *Food Chem Toxicol.* 2012 Dec 5.

61. Balansky R, Ganchev G, Iltcheva M, et al. Inhibition of lung tumor development by berry extracts in mice exposed to cigarette smoke. *Int J Cancer.* 2012;131(9):1991-7.

62. Valcheva-Kuzmanova SV, Belcheva A. Current knowledge of Aronia melanocarpa as a medicinal plant. *Folia Med (Plovdiv).* 2006;48(2):11-7.

63. Heller HJ, Greer LG, Haynes SD, Poindexter JR, Pak CY. Pharmacokinetic and pharmacodynamic comparison of two calcium supplements in postmenopausal women. *J Clin Pharmacol.* 2000;40(11):1237-44.

64. Stechschulte SA, Kirsner RS, Federman DG. Vitamin D: bone and beyond, rationale and recommendations for supplementation. *Am J Med.* 2009;122(9):793-802.

65. Holick MF. The role of vitamin D for bone health and fracture prevention. *Curr Osteoporos Rep.* 2006;4(3):96-102.

66. Holick MF. Optimal vitamin D status for the prevention and treatment of osteoporosis. *Drugs Aging.* 2007;24(12):1017-29.

67. Bügel S. Vitamin K and bone health in adult humans. *Vitam Horm.* 2008;78:393-416.

68. Bolton-Smith C, McMurdo ME, Paterson CR, et al. Two-year randomized controlled trial of vitamin K1 (phylloquinone) and vitamin D3 plus calcium on the bone health of older women. *J Bone Miner Res.* 2007;22(4):509-19.

69. Nordin BE. Calcium and osteoporosis. *Nutrition.* 1997;13(7-8):664-86.

70. Cashman KD. Calcium intake, calcium bioavailability and bone health. *Br J Nutr.* 2002;87 Suppl 2:S169-77.

71. Ryder KM, Shorr RI, Bush AJ, et al. Magnesium intake from food and supplements is associated with bone mineral density in healthy older white subjects. *J Am Geriatr Soc.* 2005;53(11):1875-80.

72. Rude RK, Singer FR, Gruber HE. Skeletal and hormonal effects of magnesium deficiency. *J Am Coll Nutr.* 2009;28(2):131-41.

73. Hyun TH, Barrett-Connor E, Milne DB. Zinc intakes and plasma concentrations in men with osteoporosis: the Rancho Bernardo Study. *Am J Clin Nutr.* 2004;80(3):715-21.

74. Lowe NM, Lowe NM, Fraser WD, Jackson MJ. Is there a potential therapeutic value of copper and zinc for osteoporosis? *Proc Nutr Soc.* 2002;61(2):181-5.

75. Bae YJ, Kim MH. Manganese supplementation improves mineral density of the spine and femur and serum osteocalcin in rats. *Biol Trace Elem Res.* 2008l;124(1):28-34.

76. Nielsen FH. Studies on the relationship between boron and magnesium which possibly affects the formation and maintenance of bones. *Magnes Trace Elem.* 1990;9(2):61-9.

77. Volpe SL, Taper LJ, Meacham S. The relationship between boron and magnesium status and bone mineral density in the human: a review. *Magnes Res.* 1993;6(3):291-6.

78. Koitaya N, Ezaki J, Nishimuta M, et al. Effect of low dose vitamin K2 (MK-4) supplementation on bio-indices in postmenopausal Japanese women. *J Nutr Sci Vitaminol* (Tokyo). 2009;55(1):15-21.

79. Iwamoto J, Takeda T, Sato Y. Role of vitamin K2 in the treatment of postmenopausal osteoporosis. *Curr Drug Saf.* 2006;1(1):87-97.

80. Chonan O, Takahashi R, Yasui H, Watanuki M. Effect of L-lactic acid on the absorption of calcium in gastrectomized rats. *J Nutr Sci Vitaminol* (Tokyo). 1998;44(6):869-75.

81. Sheikh MS, Santa Ana CA, Nicar MJ, Schiller LR, Fordtran JS. Gastrointestinal absorption of calcium from milk and calcium salts. *N Engl J Med.* 1987;317(9):532-6.

82. Jugdaohsingh R. Silicon and bone health. *J Nutr Health Aging.* 2007r;11(2):99-110.

83. Meunier PJ, Roux C, Seeman E, et al. The effects of strontium ranelate on the risk of vertebral fracture in women with postmenopausal osteoporosis. *N Engl J Med.* 2004;350(5):459-68.

84. Marie PJ, Ammann P, Boivin G, Rey C. Mechanisms of action and therapeutic potential of strontium in bone. *Calcif Tissue Int.* 2001;69(3):121-9.

85. 2. Li Z, Lu WW, Chiu PK, et al. Strontium-calcium coadministration stimulates bone matrix osteogenic factor expression and new bone formation in a large animal model. *J Orthop Res. 2009;27(6):758-62.*

86. 3. Fonseca JE. Rebalancing bone turnover in favour of formation with strontium ranelate: implications for bone strength. *Rheumatology (Oxford).* 2008;47 Suppl 4:iv17-19.

87. 1. In vitro evaluation of the effect of a specialized silica on the metabolism of bone matrix. Biopredic (Rennes, France) 1999. Data unpublished.

88. 2. A double-blind, placebo-controlled randomized study of the effect of a specialized silica on several biochemical markers of the bone remodeling. CERN (Lorient, France) 2005. Data unpublished.

89. 3. Effect of a specialized silica on osteoarticular disease and bone problems. Compilation of 150 case studies. 2006-2007. Data unpublished.

90. 4. A specialized silica for bone remineralization after trauma or for the treatment of osteoporosis. Summary of case reports. 1991-1995. Data unpublished.

91. Bremont JF. Pre- and post-treatment with Trica-Sil in dental implant patients: a review of 37 cases. Dental office (Nantes, France) 2007. Data unpublished.

92. Baliga MS, Haniadka R, Pereira MM, et al. Radioprotective effects of Zingiber officinale Roscoe (ginger): past, present and future. *Food Funct.* 2012;3(7):714-23.

93. Ryan JL, Heckler CE, Roscoe JA, et al. Ginger *(Zingiber officinale)* reduces acute chemotherapy-induced nausea: A URCC CCOP study of 576 patients. *Support Care Cancer.* 2012;20(7):1479–1489.

94. Sontakke S, Thawani V, Naik MS. Ginger as an antiemetic in nausea and vomiting induced by chemotherapy: A randomized, cross-over, double-blind study. *Indian J Pharmacol.* 2003;35:32–36.

95. Mowrey DB, Clayson DE. Motion sickness, ginger, and psychophysics. *Lancet.* 1982;1(8273):655-7.

96. Lien HC, Sun WM, Chen YH, et al. Effects of ginger on motion sickness and gastric slow-wave dysrhythmias induced by circular vection. *Am J Physiol Gastrointest Liver Physiol.* 2003 Mar;284(3):G481-9.

97. Lacasse A, Rey E, Ferreira E, Morin C, Berard A. Epidemiology of nausea and vomiting of pregnancy: prevalence, severity, determinants, and the importance of race/ethnicity. *BMC Pregnancy Childbirth.* 2009 Jul 2;9:26

98. Vutyavanich T, Kraisarin T, Ruangsri R. Ginger for nausea and vomiting in pregnancy: randomized, double-masked, placebo-controlled trial. *Obstet Gynecol.* 2001;97(4):577-82.

99. Keating A, Chez RA. Ginger syrup as an antiemetic in early pregnancy. *Altern Ther Health Med.* 2002;8(5):89-91.

100. Black CD, Herring MP, Hurley DJ, O'Connor PJ. Ginger (Zingiber officinale) reduces muscle pain caused by eccentric exercise. *J Pain.* 2010;11(9):894-903.

101. Terry R, Posadzki P, Watson LK, Ernst E. The use of ginger (Zingiber officinale) for the treatment of pain: a systematic review of clinical trials. *Pain Med.* 2011;12(12):1808-18.

102. Gruenwald J, Brendler T, Jaenicke C, eds. PDR for Herbal Medicines, 4th ed. Thomson Healthcare Inc. Montvale, NJ; 2007:365-370.

103. Xu Z, Du P, Meiser P, Jacob C. Proanthocyanidins: oligomeric structures with unique biochemical properties and great therapeutic promise. *Nat Prod Commun.* 2012;7(3):381-8.

104. Lee YA, Cho EJ, Yokozawa T. Oligomeric proanthocyanidins improve memory and enhance phosphorylation of vascular endothelial growth factor receptor-2 in senescence-accelerated mouse prone/8. *Br J Nutr.* 2010;103(4):479-89.

105. Nandakumar V, Singh T, Katiyar SK. Multi-targeted prevention and therapy of cancer by proanthocyanidins. *Cancer Lett.* 2008;269(2):378-87.

106. Bagchi D, Bagchi M, Stohs SJ, et al. Free radicals and grape seed proanthocyanidin extract: importance in human health and disease prevention. *Toxicology.* 2000;148(2-3):187-97.

107. Chacón MR, Ceperuelo-Mallafré V, Maymó-Masip E, et al. Grape-seed procyanidins modulate inflammation on human differentiated adipocytes in vitro. *Cytokine.* 2009;47(2):137-42.

108. Devaraj S, Vega-López S, Kaul N, Schönlau F, Rohdewald P, Jialal I. Supplementation with a pine bark extract rich in polyphenols increases plasma antioxidant capacity and alters the plasma lipoprotein profile. *Lipids.* 2002;37(10):931-4.

109. Koch R. Comparative study of Venostasin and Pycnogenol in chronic venous insufficiency. *Phytother Res.* 2002;16:1–5.

110. Hosseini S, Lee J, Sepulveda RT, Rohdewald P, Watson RR. A randomized, double-blind, placebo-controlled, prospective, 16 week crossover study to determine the role of Pycnogenol in modifying blood pressure in mildly hypertensive patients. *Nutr Res.* 2001;21:1251–1260.

111. Iravani S, Zolfaghari B. Pharmaceutical and nutraceutical effects of Pinus pinaster bark extract. *Res Pharm Sci.* 2011 Jan-Jun; 6(1): 1–11.

112. Ohyama K, Furuta C, et al. Catechin-rich grape seed extract supplementation attenuates diet-induced obesity in C57BL/6J mice. *Ann Nutr Metab.* 2011;58(3):250-8.

113. Charradi K, Sebai H, et al. Grape seed extract alleviates high-fat diet-induced obesity and heart dysfunction by preventing cardiac siderosis. *Cardiovasc Toxicol.* 2011;11(1):28-37.

114. Suwannaphet W, Meeprom A, Yibchok-Anun S, Adisakwattana S. Preventive effect of grape seed extract against high-fructose diet-induced insulin resistance and oxidative stress in rats. *Food Chem Toxicol.* 2010;48:1853–7.

115. Meeprom A, Sompong W, Suwannaphet W, Yibchok-Anun S, Adisakwattana S. Grape-seed extract supplementation prevents high-fructose diet-induced insulin resistance in rats by improving insulin and adiponectin signalling pathways. *Br J Nutr.* 2011;106:1173–81.

116. Be One in a Million This American Heart Month. Centers for Disease Control. Available at: http://www.cdc.gov/features/heartmonth/. Accessed on January 3, 2013.

117. Tufano A, Arturo C, Cimino E, et al. Mesoglycan: clinical evidences for use in vascular diseases. *Int J Vascular Med.* 2010; (2010); 8 pages. Article ID 390643.

118. Vecchio F, Zanchin G, Maggioni F, Santambrogio C, De Zanche L. Mesoglycan in treatment of patients with cerebral ischemia: effects on hemorheologic and hematochemical parameters. *Acta Neurol* (Napoli). 1993 Dec;15(6):449-56.

119. Caimi G, Romandini S, Lo Presti R, et al. Effect of mesoglycan on macrorheologic and microrheologic parameters. *Curr Therapeut Res.* 1992;52(3):412–418.

120. Orefice G, Troisi E, Selvaggio, et al. Effect of long-term mesoglycan treatment on fibrinogen plasma levels in patients with ischemic cerebrovascular disease. *Curr Therapeut Res.* 1992;52(5):669-670.

121. Nenci GG, Gresele P, Ferrari G, et al. Treatment of intermittent claudication with mesoglycan—a placebo-controlled, double-blind study. *Thromb Haemost.* 2001;86(5):1181-7.

122. Andreozzi GM. Effectiveness of mesoglycan in patients with previous deep venous thrombosis and chronic venous insufficiency. *Minerva Cardioangiol.* 2007 Dec;55(6):741-53.

123. Arosio E, Ferrari G, Santoro L, et al. A placebo-controlled, double-blind study of mesoglycan in the treatment of chronic venous ulcers. *Eur J Vasc Endovasc Surg.* 2001;22(4):365-72.

124. Etzel R. Special extract of Boswellia serrata in the treatment of rheumatoid arthritis. *Phytomedicine.* 1996;3(1):91-4.

125. Takahashi M. Boswellic acid exerts antitumor effects in colorectal cancer cells by modulating expression of the let-7 and miR-200 microRNA family. *Carcinogenesis.* 2012;33(12):2441-9.

126. Shen Y. Boswellic acid induces epigenetic alterations by modulating DNA methylation in colorectal cancer cells. *Cancer Bio Ther.* 2012;13(7):542-52.